Nursing Homes

How to Find a Good One
Or a Few Good Nurses in a Bad One

Frances Lovett, R.N.

Copyright © 2018 Frances Lovett, R.N.

All rights reserved.

ISBN: 1719151024
ISBN-13: 978-1719151023

IN MEMORY

OF

BILL LOVETT

CONTENTS

	Foreword	i
	Author's Note	iii
	Introduction	v
1	The Decision	1
2	Nursing Home Structure	9
3	Selection	22
4	Understanding Payment	27
5	Internet Resources	41
6	Visit	49
7	Hospital Discharge	57
8	Admission Day	74
9	Advance Directives	82
10	Resident Rights	91
11	Medications	104
12	Mealtime	119
13	Urinary Incontinence	127
14	Bowel Incontinence	135
15	Confusion	143
16	Restraints	151
17	Care Plans	159
18	Theft	169
19	Laundry	179
20	Holidays and Gifts	185
21	Advocacy	193
22	The Caregivers	209
23	Epilogue	217
	Appendix A: CMS Star Rating	221
	Appendix B: Resident's Rights	228
	Appendix C: Mealtime	234
	Acknowledgments	237
	About the Author	238

FOREWARD

You are assisting someone dear and near to you with choosing a nursing home or who already resides in a nursing home, so it is my pleasure to introduce you to Frances Lovett, author of this book. You will bless the day you opened *Nursing Homes: How to Find a Good One Or a Few Good Nurses in a Bad One*.

Frances cared for her mother in a nursing home. Frances cared for any number of cherished patients in nursing homes as their Registered Nurse and Director of Nurses. I wish it were possible to have had this information when my parents were in assisted living and nursing home facilities. Be glad that she has taken her experience in hand and offers it to all who undertake caretaking responsibility for a loved one.

You will find her your closest ally and champion. She focuses on the essential information and background needed to accomplish your work. Make no mistake, caregiving is work; it is an ultimate labor of love.

Frances speaks plainly; she discarded the extraneous information and gets to the basics. She describes succinctly each point of caregiving and follows it up with significant processes about which you need to become aware and follows up with possible traps, potholes and ditches about which you should be aware. Then, brilliantly she offers examples that bring the information home for you. She does it with love and humor to which, I testify, all caregivers need and deserve.

Read all of it. Refer to it often. Make notes for yourself in order to keep track of what you have done and must accomplish. It will become your manual and will keep you sane.

Rose M. Hall

Proud to call Frances Lovett, Friend

AUTHOR'S NOTE

A lasting impression of my nursing home experience is the emotional upset family and friends endure when an unwilling person requires nursing home admission. The new resident is often defiant—accusing loved ones of all manner of crime and ugly motives. Caring family and friends cajole, attempt to pacify and jump through hoops trying to ease the new resident's trauma. They also spend a lot of time apologizing to staff; "This is not my mother, she is really a sweet person" or "Dad has never acted this way. This foul mouth is totally out of character for him."

Many years ago I resolved to relieve my family of this emotional turmoil by giving them early permission to "haul me off." I forgave them in advance. I warned them I might be cursing, screaming, scratching, biting, kicking or spitting but that was okay. The nursing home is quite capable of handling all of the above and I will be fine. I said, "Don't worry. Get on with your life."

I did not offer this directive in a flippant or cavalier manner. I believed it. This conviction was well founded and based on my nursing home work experience.

A few years later, I altered my directive. I told my family to find me a *good* nursing home. Then they could drop me off and get on with their lives.

Today, my directive no longer stands in any form. I know that even if my family finds a good nursing home, I will still need their help and oversight of my care. This 360 degree turn is based on the reality of changes I faced as a Director of Nursing, Medicare Coordinator, clinical consultant, medical sales representative, Legal Nurse Consultant and auditor during my career. I visited hundreds of nursing homes in Texas. My lament is supported by my peers throughout the state and nationally.

The frustrating journey of trying to attain minimal nursing home care for my own mother solidified my new position. My attention has now turned to educating my family in Nursing Home 101.

My children's response to NH 101 instruction has been "Write it down. We need a manual." That was the impetus for this book. I hope it proves helpful to other children, spouses and friends as well. Selecting the right nursing home is not easy, but it is worth the effort and will be rewarded by better care for the resident and less stress for the family.

This guide follows my mother's journey and includes incidents from my daily nursing home duties. The narratives are accurate, needing no embellishment. They were lifted from notes kept in my ever-present spiral notebooks. Throughout this book I present these accounts as EXAMPLES for the BE AWARE and BEWARE sections.

Addendums and Endnotes provide additional details, references and long-term care organization contacts. At print time several referenced government websites are undergoing revisions which may become problematic for cited links. My own family's names are accurate, all others have been changed.

Sometimes accused of writing from a perspective of anger, I affirm such feelings emerge with each report of lost dignity, suffering and needless death within a nursing home. I make no apologies if objectivity seems lost because the industry as a whole makes no attempt to correct its long-standing lack of transparency or offer reliable help for those entrusted to its care . . . in spite of decades of opportunities to do so.

Frances Lovett, R.N.

INTRODUCTION

My thirty year association with nursing homes began in central Texas. It involved, among other things, employment as a staff nurse and Director of Nursing. In early years the industry was characterized by local ownership and emphasis was usually on patient care. Focus on care gave way to profit margins as national corporations foresaw vast amounts of money to be made.

As this change was taking place, I transitioned into consulting and saw the effects of the shift in emphasis on nursing homes statewide. The totality of facilities I entered should have revealed a significant number of conscientious homes providing good patient care. It did not. Instead, the miniscule number delivering even minimal care was discouraging.

My experience in Texas exposed the calamity of nursing home care in the state, and revealed the barriers to finding a good nursing home. It is the stuff of comedy except for the tragedy brought to those dependent upon the industry. I was soon to discover that the care does not get any better outside the state.

As a legal nurse consultant for nursing home litigation, I reviewed medical records from facilities across the country. They revealed the same dismal conditions. Professional networking with peers in other states confirmed corresponding situations in overwhelming numbers.

Navigating the delicate and painful decisions of nursing home placement often leaves loved ones, family and friends feeling lost, helpless and vulnerable. Choices are made more difficult by an absence of meaningful resources. Confusing information and unanswered questions can leave anyone attempting to compare facilities feeling frustrated and alone.

The sole purpose of this guide is to provide help. Still, the journey will not be easy given the industry's control and mindset. Limited choices in some locations and financial obstacles will prove to be further hurdles for some.

The aim of each consumer, family member or friend, will always be to locate a good nursing home. This guide will assist you in identifying one of those special nursing homes. It will also prepare you for the more likely alternative of having to rely upon a few good nurses in a bad nursing home. Even in the worst of circumstances you should find enough information to take control of your loved one's care and rights.

Not only have I walked in your shoes with my own loved ones, my association with the industry provides insight into the dilemmas faced by every nursing home consumer.

Families and new patients struggle with nursing home selection, the admission process and daily facility routine. This guide will help you recognize the doubletalk, red flags and shenanigans nursing homes throw at you along the way and then it provides a path forward for attaining your loved one's best interest.

I also hope you gain a fresh appreciation for the untold value of our nursing home population—their life experiences, contributions, honesty and humor.

Frances Lovett, R.N.

CHAPTER 1

THE DECISION

If you struggle with the decision to seek nursing home care for yourself or a loved one, you are not alone. Many cross the troubling waters into nursing home care every day and the future holds boatloads more. Strong currents often push against that choice: promises ("I'll never put you in a nursing home"), rejection by the patient, disagreement among family members, finances and legal issues.

Ideally, nursing home admission is a collaborative effort between the patient, family, friends and physician. Such harmony is seldom the case. Nursing homes' dismal reputation only makes matters worse.

Love and respect for a family member can delay nursing home care while common threads weave into a patchwork of stressors: safety, personal hygiene and twenty-four-hour oversight. It is rare for the person needing nursing home care to agree with the move.

Friends want to help but prefer to remain on the sideline because they share the same fears as their friend needing the care. Physicians are not much help until there is a medical event such as a broken hip or stroke.

The nursing home decision eventually rests with the patient and his or her family. Spouses typically struggle to keep their loved one at home long after recognizing the need for nursing home admission. It is not unusual for the caregiving spouse's health to decline as they become physically and mentally exhausted, sometimes needing nursing home care themselves.

Often adult children begin the awkward transition toward parenting their parents with the realization that around-the-clock care is needed. Doubtful gray areas arise, especially if a parent does not agree. Gray fades into transparency over time, often after attempting help at home and in assisted living facilities. A hospitalization can clarify the decision.

Nursing homes seem more acceptable when labeled skilled nursing facilities, care centers, nursing centers or rehabilitation centers (distinguish from acute rehabilitation centers). Whatever the packaging, arriving at the decision to seek nursing home placement is a milestone and even more so when the elder agrees.

In the BE AWARE and BEWARE sections you will find a few factors influencing the decision for nursing home care. EXAMPLES follow and you will soon be able to add your own unique story. Subsequent chapters provide information on selecting a nursing home and nuances of admission and care.

BE AWARE
- Very few new residents have accepted the nursing home as a permanent arrangement when they arrive.
- Instances of couples with one spouse, or sometimes both, needing twenty-four-hour care present double trouble, especially if both are determined to "die at home." Typically, each adds support to the other's decision.
- In the instance of couples or family caregivers, financial obstacles sometimes enter the picture. Social Security and retirement checks will be funneled to the nursing home, thus leaving those remaining at home with a financial loss. Family members who are not dependent upon the elder's checks often face resistance from family members needing the Social Security check's income.
- Role reversal (children caring for parents), although difficult, is a factor in most nursing home admissions.
- Children living a distance from parents are at a disadvantage in recognizing a parent's decline and need for twenty-four-hour oversight.
- The elderly usually recognize their own decline in physical and mental abilities. Even so, they tend to isolate themselves at home, gradually shutting out regular contacts or anyone who might recognize and report their worsening condition.
- Disagreement among family members, especially children, is a major obstacle to a resident's acceptance of nursing home care and settling in after admission.
- In-home care is often attempted but dependable staffing and costs present mounting problems, especially when managing from a distance.

BEWARE
- A person cannot be admitted to a nursing home against their will unless declared incompetent, which usually involves a physician and court determination.
- Physicians may not recognize the need for nursing home care. They only see their patient in the office or clinical setting and cannot comprehend their struggles at home. Above all, physicians avoid declaring someone incompetent. They associate such determinations with legal entanglements.
- Some families approach the nursing home in tears after secure retirements and even fortunes have been squandered by a confused or vulnerable elder. In some cases the extent of the financial and emotional damage is not realized until after nursing home admission.

EXAMPLE: A family's failed attempt for nursing home care.

The eighty-five-year-old rancher's arrival at the nursing home was troubling. After three days in the hospital her injuries were painfully visible: deep bruises of her face and neck; swollen, purple eyelids bulged from her eye sockets leaving her barely able to see; a splint and sling hanging from her neck protected broken bones in her right arm and shoulder.

Staff slid her as gently as possible from the ambulance stretcher to the bed, still she screamed in agony. Further examination revealed bruises, scratches and swelling of her body and legs. A line of sutures on her left thigh attested to a significant gash. The hospital reported her injuries were caused by a fall and noted she was intoxicated when EMS brought her to the emergency room.

Two sons, her only family, lived in remote cities. Each questioned Mother about her plans to return to the rugged Hill Country Ranch. For most of the year she was the only human on the large spread. She managed her herd of cattle with seasonal hired help. The nearest town was an hour's drive away.

Her sons' concerns for her safety and isolation were ignored. She remained steadfast in her plans to return to the ranch. At last the frustrated eldest son said, "Mother, they said you were drunk when you got to the emergency room."

She screamed, "You're all a bunch of damn teetotalers! What the hell do you know about being drunk?"

Within two weeks she could feed herself and manage a few personal chores with her awkward left hand. She took a few unsteady steps with a cane. Mother rejected both sons' reasonable request, "Just stay a couple of weeks until you can walk better."

Without legal authority or a declaration of incompetence, her sons had no leverage. They did refuse to help her get back to the ranch. She called a neighboring rancher to drive her home and refused the help of home health nurses. The exasperated sons assured staff they would attempt some kind of oversight, perhaps with the rancher she trusted.

EXAMPLE: A daughter's painful decisions for nursing home care.

Mother and daughter breezed through the stressful admission process. Both answered the nurse's health questions while the daughter organized drawers, hung clothes and arranged personal articles in the bedside stand. Mother and daughter bantered back and forth as though they were back home in the kitchen.

Within thirty minutes, the mother seemed pleased with her room and nursing staff understood the care she needed. Although alert and talkative, all her movement was limited by arthritis. She needed assistance to get out of bed, walk to the bathroom, bathe and with personal hygiene.

They described an efficient home routine with one warning from the daughter, "If she calls needing to get to the bathroom, you'd better send your fastest runner." They enjoyed a chuckle while recalling the consequences of a recent slow response by the daughter.

The daughter visited daily, usually early morning or late evening. She helped staff fix snafus with Mother's laundry, food and nursing routine. During a rare afternoon visit, I found her sitting alone while staff showered Mother. She seemed tired and worried.

"Is there anything we can do to make Mother's stay easier for you?" I asked.

"Oh no. I just feel so bad. I'd like to take her home. My husband misses her conversation. We were fine for six years then my father had a stroke. My parents divorced thirty years ago. Mother stayed in San Antonio and Dad moved to Austin. Now he's in a skilled nursing facility. He's not alert like Mother and I'm totally responsible for him. Neither of them remarried and I'm their only child.

"I must check on him every day because of problems with his care. I spend most of my time running up and down I-35 between San Antonio and Austin. On most days, I barely get to see my husband. I've thought about moving Dad to San Antonio, but it doesn't seem fair to move him away from his home, friends and doctors. I couldn't leave Mother alone all day and that's why I brought her here. We've talked about our situation. She understands, but it's still hard not having her at home. I'm hoping Dad improves and his care gets better, then I won't need to go so often."

I could only assure her that staff would watch Mother closely and call if we noticed any changes. I encouraged her to consider substituting a call to the nurses for a visit, especially when she's short on time. Hopefully, she would gain enough confidence in Mother's care to ease the burden of daily visits.

EXAMPLE: My family's attempt at damage control as our mother's dementia progressed.

Following my father's death, a circle of close friends provided Mother's support system for forty years. Her retirement income from the school cafeteria, Social Security and oil royalties assured a comfortable life in the small town of Powell, Wyoming. Nevertheless, she insisted on working at the local bowling alley into her seventies.

In her early eighties Mother began describing falls and bruises when I called. She was forgetful and repetitive during our conversations.

My sister Jean made regular trips from Cheyenne. She always found the cabinets and refrigerator empty and her house a mess. She cried over the food-stained clothes Mother wore, but could not find clean ones. She bought Mother new clothes which never made it to the wash.

Mother isolated herself from old friends, making them feel unwelcome. She preferred the company of teenagers and young adults. Family contacts reported some of the youths to be unsavory and unknown to the community.

During one call, Mother laughed, "Sometimes I wake up with kids I don't even know sleeping all over my living room floor." Neighbors confirmed her overnight guests.

Mother was defiant and hostile as the family moved through gentle, loving and then frank attempts to move her toward 24-hour supervision. Her emotions and accusations intensified. "You're just trying to take me away from my friends."

On a visit, I found three young adults embedded in the house, even though, she expected our arrival. Mother's anxiety accelerated as they gathered their belongings and left. She seemed "mixed up" to my son.

Finding no food in the house, I asked her to drive me to get take-out chicken. Thoughts of evaluating her mental capacity vanished into my own psychological angst with Mother speeding, running stop signs and being generally obnoxious behind the wheel. I questioned, "Mother aren't you afraid of wrecking or killing somebody?"

"Everybody in town knows my old Plymouth, they can just get the hell out of the way." On the return home, she circled the same familiar landmarks several times—lost in daylight just three blocks from home.

I guided her homeward. "Mother, I'm worried about you driving at night. Are you sure you could find your way home?"

"I don't need to drive at night. I have friends I can call."

I invited her to join us on a jaunt through Yellowstone Park. She refused. "You're just trying to take me away from my friends."

Her long-time physician rejected our request for a determination of incompetence. He said, "I think she's doing pretty good. After all, she still gets around town and enjoys her friends." His documentation of incompetence was necessary for us to pursue legal oversight.

An agreement to visit an assisted living facility near Jean's home culminated in a defiant bus ride back to Powell; she wrecked a family Christmas with behavioral antics; family attempts to discuss her safety initiated bitter, foul cursing; and all conversations circled back to accusations of interference with her friends—the overnight youth. Rudeness and anger toward Jean escalated with each exhausting four-hour drive to restock groceries, clean her house and take care of laundry.

"I don't want you here. I've got friends," she told Jean. Sometimes, Mother refused to talk at all.

Jean's husband Dick was Mother's medical power of attorney. A native son of Powell, he knew her physician. A social worker by profession, he gathered data he felt would convince the doctor of her incompetence and need for oversight. Dick's efforts gleaned a slight concession from the doctor, "She might need a little help." He would not contribute to any incompetence effort. Attorneys were sympathetic but unable to intervene as they interpreted Wyoming law.

The family agreed to step back, treat her with love, but no longer visit her in Powell or offer support to her erratic behavior.

Dick was also Mother's financial power of attorney. Through the years he filed her taxes, handled her monthly expenses, credit card overcharges and bank overdrafts. Several years previously, he reduced her to one credit card, negotiated her debt with the local banker and schooled her on a budget. She managed with only a few mishaps for several years. We did not approve of how she spent money, but agreed it was hers to spend as she chose.

During a roaring blizzard Jean received Mother's tearful call, "Please send me some money. They're going to turn off my power if I don't pay my bill. The bank won't take my checks."

"Mother, I'll bring you to my house while we arrange for assisted living. I won't send you any money."

"Okay!" Mother shouted.

She tried to disrupt plans as facility arrangements moved forward by calling friends seeking a ride back to Powell. She wrangled to move into Jean's home instead of the facility. After admission, adult grandchildren and friends learned to turn a deaf ear to bribery attempts in her relentless efforts to return to Powell.

Dick's unraveling of her finances revealed debts traceable to youthful friends, a co-signed bank note for a pick-up truck in default, her credit card maxed out with liquor and convenience store charges and her checks to local merchants returned as insufficient funds. The pharmacist, a family friend, believed her tearful explanations of not having enough money for medications. He continued filling her prescriptions in spite of months of unpaid charges.

Mother settled into assisted living. She enjoyed her new friends and activities. Confusion worsened and outbursts of anger toward

Jean continued. Later, Jean and Dick relocated to Reno, Nevada and transferred Mother to a nearby assisted living facility. Her adjustment proved to be rocky. She often refused to eat, bathe or leave her room. We had previously agreed that Jean's responsibility would be assisted living; my oversight would begin when mother needed nursing home care. I made arrangements for her admission to a San Antonio nursing home.

Mother did not resist the limited information we provided—only that she was moving to a new home in Texas. We agreed that further detail would cause added confusion and anxiety without any possibility of changing course. I'm sure she did not understand what was happening.

She engaged fellow passengers in charming stories on the flight from Reno. During a bathroom visit one commented, "She's really doing well for a ninety-five-year-old."

I chuckled and shook my head. "She's really only eighty-seven and you wouldn't believe the rest of the story."

Mother returned to her seat as the descent into San Antonio began. My thoughts nosedived into preparation for the next few hours. How would Mother react to finally arriving at a nursing home?

EXAMPLE: Strategies used to delay and evade the decision for twenty-four-hour care.

As a home health nurse I often found a husband and wife managing in a situation where one is mentally competent but physically debilitated and their spouse is physically fit but mentally impaired. They had moved into a symbiotic mode with one giving instructions and the other dutifully obeying: cook, wash, clean the house, etc. Thus both are kept on an even keel, but in the absence of either, due perhaps to hospitalization or death, the family or responsible party must face the reality of twenty-four-hour care.

The mentally competent, but physically impaired may struggle beyond their capacity to survive even with the usual community supports such as Meals on Wheels and home health care. They may decide to shut down outside contacts if they become suspicious that caregivers are guiding them toward nursing home admission.

CHAPTER 2

NURSING HOME STRUCTURE

Shopping for a nursing home is never pleasant. Most consider it a chore unpleasant enough to delay until an urgent need arises, thus leaving us vulnerable to misinformation and salesmanship. Choosing the best nursing home requires maneuvering through a minefield of contradictions, complexities and pseudo-authorities. However, obtaining your own facts allows you to separate truth from slick marketing techniques, sort out quality options and arrive at an informed decision.

Expect to achieve greater insight than your conversations with nursing home and hospital employees provide. Their knowledge is often limited to the narrow scope of their employer's training and interest. A broader insight into the vast nursing home industry is rewarded by saved time and resources, fewer mistakes, less stress and comfortable self-confidence.

I suggest mastering the ambiguous vocabulary and then move on to the nursing home structure: ownership, operation and residents. Hopefully, this chapter will serve as a quick reference with succeeding chapters offering the detail you need.

VOCABULARY

The **long-term care industry** and the **nursing home industry** are both expansive commercial enterprises.

Long-term care is an umbrella term referring to institutions providing clients service over an extended period of time. Nursing homes, assisted living, residential care complexes, and boarding homes are a few examples of the long-term care industry.

Nursing home industry refers to the part of long-term care we call nursing homes and all of the varied commercial interests associated with each facility. Contracts between nursing homes, big pharmaceutical interests, food service giants, medical equipment manufacturers, rehabilitation services, office, cleaning and medical supply companies are the norm. A mix of national, regional and local contracts include consultants for nursing, medical records, billing and technical support. Nationwide real estate brokers, investors and management companies are unseen but ever present in facility decisions. A few local vendors are used for lawn service, small repairs, fresh produce and odd jobs. Most employees within the building are hired locally and the nursing home payroll contributes significantly to a small community's economy.

Quality of care is a vague term claiming excellence in the care a nursing home provides. Further descriptions add individualized, loving, caring, personal and other affectionate terms to define quality of care. Claims are often based on results of the last inspection. Passing a state nursing home inspection simply means the facility met minimum standards on the day of inspection. Sometimes, facilities erroneously quote regulations in order to limit service. Nursing homes who provide quality of care realize their responsibility goes beyond rules and regulations to include resident requests and comfort. True quality of care is evidenced by a facility's focus on resident kindness and respect. Such a facility's boundary for resident care is the health and safety of each resident and staff member, not inspections and regulations. There is no conflict between quality care and nursing home regulations.

A **skilled nursing facility** (SNF: s-n-i-f) is a nursing home. Skilled nursing facility sounds more palatable than *nursing home* or the archaic *rest home,* thus the industry uses it as a marketing tool. Other terms include nursing center, care center, nursing and rehabilitation center, health center, health and rehabilitation center or any combination of these terms. I use **nursing home** throughout this book because the term is universally understood.

Like restaurants, nursing homes are inspected by each states' department of health and issued a license to provide service consistent with consumer protections. You will find the license for both establishments displayed in a prominent place. The restaurant license ensures every customer the same sanitation and food standards. The license to operate a skilled nursing facility (nursing home) guarantees every customer (resident) the same skilled nursing care.

Skilled nursing care means nursing services given or supervised by licensed nurses: RN (registered nurse), LVN (licensed vocational nurse), LPN (licensed practical nurse). Every client within the building is entitled to the same skilled nursing care just as every restaurant customer is entitled to the same sanitation and food standards.

Marketers hawk their **skilled unit** as providing superior care. In truth, such care is no better than any other care within the building. The often dubbed **Medicare skilled** distinction means the lucrative Medicare program is being billed for care received on this unit also, another misnomer, because residents with other payment sources are usually on the same unit. The distinct Medicare skilled units are set up to shift facility expenses into the annual Medicare cost report—high salaries, therapy expenditures and square footage. Some facilities have deserted the Medicare skilled unit concept and admit Medicare residents to beds throughout the building. The concept benefits residents by avoiding the hassle and stress of moving to another room when Medicare payment ends.

A **hospital skilled nursing** unit does not deliver better skilled care than a local nursing home even though hospital social workers and discharge planners selectively recommend their own skilled unit for the most profitable Medicare patients.

The designation of **for-profit** versus **not-for-profit** is a deceptive notion within the nursing home business. All nursing homes require a profit for survival. A very few turn profits back into the nursing home for resident benefit. Not-for-profits use their profits in the same ways as for-profits: management fees, administrative bonuses and capital improvements; hence, arriving at zero profit. For-profits also show very little or no profit and maybe even losses.

Chains refers to two or more nursing homes linked together by the same corporate ownership. They usually include multiple facilities spread across states, regions and the entire country. Increasing percentages of revenue spent on administration and management and decreasing percentages spent on resident care are characteristic of chain-operated facilities.

Patient, client, and **resident** are all recycled references to nursing home occupants. The term, **resident**, prevails today because of widespread efforts to create a home-like environment, hinting of a place where you can live happily for a long time.

STRUCTURE

Nursing homes are more complex than meets the eye. Layers of organizational structure have a direct affect on each resident. Within this structure the pursuit of quality care often seems elusive. Yet, we need not sacrifice expectations of quality care for our loved ones. Understanding the three moving parts of every facility (ownership, operations, residents) enhances chances of success.

Ownership of nursing homes runs the gamut of proprietorships from private individuals owning one facility, to regional and national chains owning multiple facilities. There are many financial structures including trusts, churches, hospitals, charitable-groups, government and combined organizational structures. There is a recent trend of nursing homes partnering with hospitals. The reasoning is that plaintiffs' attorneys are less likely to bring legal action when hospitals are involved.

Management companies are layered between corporate owners and individual facilities, sometimes several for each nursing home. Every management company is on the receiving end of management fees assessed to the individual nursing homes. The same names seem to crop up in the corporations and the management companies' boards and officers.

Ownership free of chain control does not guarantee better care, but identifying ownership provides a hint of the operating philosophy and where the money goes, i.e., resident care or hidden profit margins. You can be sure large national chains will place heavy emphasis on profits.

Operations within each nursing home determine the mood, quality of care and value placed on each resident. It is by far the most important segment and warrants an objective look at the **administrator** and **director of nurses.** You may encounter more creative titles such as Chief Operating Executive, Director of Patient Services, Chief Nursing Executive, etc. In the fluid environment of nursing home employment the two often travel in tandem from one facility to another. They run the nursing home. When either or both change, the care may improve or get worse.

Volatility characterizes the dynamics of nursing home structure. Frequent resignations, terminations and travel between buildings for better pay, bonuses and career advancement are the norm. Often this upheaval is necessitated by corporate sales or changes in management companies. The administrator or nursing director may resign because of conflicting philosophy or new management's reputation for bad care. New ownership usually prefers their own administrator and nursing director—well indoctrinated, proven stewards of the corporation's objectives. Each change creates unrest for staff and their residents, therefore the tenure of administrative staff is a good indicator of stability within the nursing home. Non-chain owned facilities usually afford more permanent management.

Administrators set the tone and focus within each building by finessing their way through regulatory compliance, building maintenance and the budget. Expenditures within the building are tied to incoming revenue, i.e., the number of occupied beds in the building. Chain ownership often involves daily reports transmitted to a central office where penny pinchers control everyday expenditures. Empty beds mean less revenue and nursing staff hours is the first sacrificial offering toward a balanced daily budget.

A few insightful administrators are creative in maintaining nursing staff hours. They understand that poor resident care is the predictable result of cuts in nursing assistants' and nurses' hours. Administrators working for non-chain owners usually have greater flexibility because they work from a monthly budget and are free from daily reporting and oversight.

Directors of nursing determine the quality of resident care through staffing, oversight and policies. The position carries the huge responsibilities of delivering individualized nursing care to divergent residents and establishing staff attitude and performance. The nursing budget weighs heavily in determining how many nurses and nursing assistants are available for meeting these objectives. Effective directors of nursing devote long hours of hard work under stressful conditions, understanding they have a job rather than a position.

Residents contribute to the tenor of any nursing home. Their local mores set the mood for décor, holiday festivities, religious influences, food choices, staff approaches and the overall pace of the building. Some nursing homes offer specialized care for conditions such as dementia, wounds, strokes, psychiatry and other problems; their residents reflect these characteristics.

Residents' payment sources are evidenced by the surroundings in each nursing home but the universal expectation of quality care resonates across financial and cultural variances.

Many nuances and your questions regarding care will be explored in succeeding chapters. The focus will be on the challenges and approaches to securing the best care for you or your loved one. The BE AWARE sections provide additional detail and BEWARE indicates cautionary situations. Subsequent EXAMPLES attempt further clarification.

BE AWARE

- During the early 1990s, ownership of individual nursing homes began shifting from locally owned private, church, city and county operations to regional and national chains. By the end of that decade, venture capital groups mixed with management companies. The aging population with their guaranteed revenue stream of Medicare and Medicaid seemed limitless. Nursing home building and acquisitions accelerated resulting in a changed landscape for nursing home consumers and employees.
- The last statistics available from the Center for Disease Control show 55.7 percent of nursing homes were chain affiliated in 2014. The Kaiser Foundation set the national percentage at 50 percent chain ownership in 2011.
- Most chains lease their facility buildings from a real estate investment trust (REIT). Even though changes in the property's ownership may go unannounced, sales and real estate values figure into operations and expenditures for each nursing home, affecting the bottom line, and thus, patient care. Often REIT investors include executives from the management company operating the nursing home.
- Investment in capital improvements is advantageous for tax purposes and resale value of the building. Labor and resident comfort items are operating expenses subject to the budget's goal of profit.
- Employees call the worst of situations, "Bleeding us to death." The reference is to a new owner's tactic of draining all incoming revenue into corporate coffers. Dollars are cut from staffing, supply and food budgets; only emergency repairs are authorized and invoices go unpaid. The result is predictable: bad care, inspection deficiencies, fines, bankruptcy and a fire sale price for the dilapidated facility. Good nursing homes with good revenue streams are prime targets for such schemes.
- The combination of corporate ownership, multiple management companies and REITs creates a tangle of secrecy and defensive legal barriers designed to protect the network of corporations from consumer inquiries and plaintiffs' attorneys.
- Headquarters for most large chains are located in Delaware, the state offering corporations the most legal protection against regulatory fines, litigation and financial responsibility.

- The Affordable Care Act moved the industry toward more ownership transparency, but pinning down liability for resident care remains elusive.
- Nursing homes actively support their well-established state and national trade organizations. Their lobbyists have carried considerable influence with legislators and legislation for many years.
- Within recent years consumer advocacy groups have organized and proven to be relentless in their efforts to change resident care for the better. Their influence is noteworthy in advancing improvements in residents' rights and quality of care measures. In September 2016, The Center for Medicare and Medicaid Services (CMS) began implementing the most comprehensive rule revisions since 1991. However, the incoming administration placed many of the revisions on hold beginning in 2018.

BEWARE
- Contrary to promotions, a **religious** affiliation or name is not a predictor of better care but is more often another publicity ploy.
- Determining ownership may be impossible. A building's façade and public information usually leads one to envision a local enterprise, but the real ownership is often disguised. Most large chains organize each facility to look like an independent operation accountable for their own financial and legal decisions, even though the distant management company rules over any significant action within the facility: staffing, maintenance, budget.

EXAMPLE: Two facilities organized and promoted as individual operations, but owned by the same corporation.

After resigning my position at a San Antonio nursing home, I received notice of the facility's Chapter 11 bankruptcy from the U.S. Bankruptcy Court. The court action was in progress during my employment, but the nursing home had not notified their employees of the bankruptcy. I received notification because my resignation triggered the Court letter informing me of my right to enter financial claims into the proceedings.

Long after Mother became a resident in a rural nursing home some distance from San Antonio, I looked through her admission paperwork while trying to find the procedure for filing a complaint with the corporate ownership. Small print revealed the same Louisiana address as listed on the Bankruptcy Court papers.

My employment and Mother's nursing home stay coincided for months, yet this was my first hint of any connection between the two facilities. The same corporate ownership explained why Mother endured the same problems as residents in the San Antonio location—short staffing, limited supplies, laundry problems, staff turnover and medication problems to name a few.

EXAMPLE: A nursing home administrator's struggle with management fees.

A trusted nursing home administrator once confided her frustration to me. I was her director of nurses.

"This company is really low-down sorry. I can't put any of my profits back into the improvements we need. I like to run a good nursing home and make money at the same time. I always show some profit at the end of the month but the management company just adjusts their fees upward every month to the amount of my profit. Of course, this is in addition to the monthly fee already figured into my budget. The monthly charge is always there! I just get charged an additional fee, the amount of that month's profit."

This company illustrates the worst of ownership—one of the largest national chains with corporate offices located in Delaware. Our rural facility's public impression was of a vague individual owner in Houston. The nursing home's misleading name was a diversion from the complex layers of management and investment groups structured to shield from any financial or legal responsibility while draining every possible penny of revenue.

We understood the implications of our facility's venture capital structure: barriers to resident care, the possibility of bankruptcy resulting in new ownership at any time and our questionable employment with any new owners. We also realized the likelihood that new proprietorship would simply mean a new facility name with the same corporate faces and a new Delaware address.

EXAMPLE: An administrator's explanation of bankruptcy and ownership change.

 A prominent new sign was the first hint of trouble as I drove into the San Antonio nursing home's parking lot. It identified the familiar building by a different name and new ownership. I visited this facility frequently as a nursing consultant. The change happened quickly.
 A national contract between the nursing home corporation and my employer paid for consultation, beds and therapeutic mattresses, when their residents needed treatment for bedsores. A number of invoices remained unpaid after several months of billing. I hoped a gentle reminder to the administrator, George, would assure payment. He always seemed amiable and in tight control of the building's operations.
 As usual, I checked the condition of the resident requiring our service before reporting to his office. He always expected a written report on progress and an estimate of how long the resident would require our added expense. He was not interested in his report today.
 "Those invoices in your hand aren't gonna get paid, so don't get me agitated by asking about 'em."
 George sported a new, oversized name tag and title identifying him as Regional Director. I congratulated him on his promotion and asked about the new sign.
 "Well, you know how it is, Frances. It's really the same company and the same people. They just went into bankruptcy, reorganized, bought it back, and changed the name. You're lucky, Frances. You work for a Fortune 500 company. You'll get your paycheck. What about the local vendors going broke because they're never going to get paid?" The young executive chuckled and twisted in his swivel chair.
 "George, I don't understand. What do you mean local vendors?"
 "Oh you know, the fresh produce guy, electrician, plumber, yard guy." He raised his arms in a helpless gesture. "Our corporation's nursing homes were their main customer and in some cases their only customer. When the corporation sold all eight of their San Antonio

facilities, those little guys lost all their customers and they all had a stack of unpaid invoices just like yours."

"Now George, you said 'sold'. I thought it was bankruptcy."

"Frances, it doesn't matter. Nobody's going to get paid. Those guys are just out of business."

George presented the stark reality of a national corporation executing a successful venture capital plan. This Delaware-based corporation enjoyed status as the largest provider of nursing home care in Texas, whether based on actual patient count or the number of facilities owned. Their Texas model of owning most of the rural nursing homes and a competitive number in urban markets existed across the country.

Their third bankruptcy in as many years remained largely unnoticed nationally. However, staff, families and residents of each facility were keenly aware of the impact on their care. The merry-go-round produced near intolerable variances in staffing, nursing care, supplies, food deliveries, utilities, repairs and state inspections.

EXAMPLE: How two administrators operating under the same ownership influenced their facilities differently.

A not-for-profit trust owned and operated two facilities in the city. One facility located in an elite economic district seemed to be a mess. The anxious administrator wasted time wrangling over national contract pricing which we could not alter. Nursing staff was ever changing and I rarely saw residents enjoying the exquisitely decorated common areas. There were many empty rooms in the building.

The second facility located across town in a less prestigious neighborhood presented a different picture. The building was vibrant with interaction between staff and residents maneuvering through cats, dogs, birdcages and aquariums. Most importantly, staff responded to every resident's need whether requested or simply observed. Nurses employed there for years lovingly protected their residents from any discomfort. Contract pricing never slowed the administrator's decision to provide needed medical equipment. He enjoyed the luxury of a waiting list for any empty beds.

I felt compelled to compliment the administrator on my pleasurable experience of consulting in his facility. He lamented, "Thank you, Frances, but I'm really worried. Our board of directors recently changed from little blue-haired ladies to young businessmen and accountants. I'm not sure my profit margins will be enough for them."

EXAMPLE: A small scale operation showing hidden ownership and management.

"Frances you won't believe what I just saw! You won't believe it! I can't believe my own eyes!" The volume of my colleague's voice was deafening, even over my cell phone. Beverly's rant continued. "I'm sitting in the parking lot at Loving Care Center watching Albert and Edwin unload a U-Haul truck full of office furniture."
Enough said.
We were familiar with the congenial brothers, Albert and Edwin Angleton. They purchased our company's mattresses for their small group of nursing homes in the Rio Grande Valley. Soon after delivery the nursing homes' licenses to operate were revoked. A rare Department of Health ruling prohibited the brothers from further participation in nursing home operations in Texas. The expected bankruptcy ensued, and mattress invoices were never paid.
Beverly shouted, "Frances, something's wrong! This stinks to high heaven. They're setting up an office inside Loving Care Center!"
As nurses, we worked for a manufacturer of therapeutic beds and mattresses. Typically, we received calls from facilities needing help because a state inspector cited them for resident bedsores or they expected such trouble on an upcoming inspection.
A string of previous owners with poor credit ratings and bankruptcies meant our corporate office denied any service to Loving Care Center. Mrs. Jordan, the new owner, called describing her dire circumstances. "I just took over this building. The state's given me one week to show improvement in the bedsores."
In the absence of a credit history for Mrs. Jordan and the presence of her urgent need, our corporate office approved credit and allowed a contract with Loving Care Center. Therapeutic mattresses were delivered. I spent long hours providing staff instruction and assistance for their many residents with bedsores. State inspectors were gradually lifting threats of sanctions as residents' bedsores improved.

I asked the Director of Nursing, "Why isn't Mrs. Jordan ever in the building?"

"Well, she's just here when we need something signed. Albert takes care of everything else."

A more intense credit check revealed Mrs. Jordan to be the Angleton's niece and the owner of record only. A totally different surname misled anyone anticipating placement of a resident at the facility, potential employees and providers of necessary services such as food, supplies and oxygen equipment. Both the Texas Department of Health, who issued the nursing home license, and our corporate office had been conned.

Beds and consultations continued until the bedsores healed. The invoices were never paid although the facility reaped considerable revenue from Medicare and Medicaid through our efforts.

References

A CDC publication from 2016 provides a comprehensive overview of the long-term care industry with nursing home statistics.
http://www.cdc.gov/nchs/data/series/sr_03/sr03_038.pdf

CDC ownership data from 2017:
www.cdc.gov/nchs/fastats/nursing-home-care.htm

CHAPTER 3

SELECTION

I wish I could assure that the decision for nursing home care ends stress for you and your loved one. Experience with my mother's nursing home care, and attempts to help other families and residents, attests to a never-ending need for vigilance, problem solving and advocacy. The intent of this chapter is to provide an overview of the first problem, selecting a nursing home.

Choosing a nursing home is not an easy process, but more often, a time consuming burden. When uncertainties challenge your physical stamina and emotional resolve, it is helpful to rely on your common sense. Answers become more evident with each inquiry made, often through a process of elimination.

Payment methods may limit choices. However, remain confident because you determine where your resources are used, whether Medicare, Medicaid, long-term care insurance, private payment or a combination of these options.

Availability will impact your choices. Urban areas offer a wide variety of choices, but rural areas are often limited to one or two nursing homes within driving distance. For families scattered across the country, selection may involve a deeper decision—relocate the loved one near a family member or oversee nursing home care from a distance.

Expect contradictory information (advertising versus government data) to test your good judgment. Internet search results, including state and federal websites, are improving but do not always provide the trustworthy facts needed for side-by-side comparisons.

What if a hospital says that your loved one will be discharged within twenty-four hours, needs a skilled nursing facility and you haven't begun your search?

Rest assured, all of the above obstacles can be overcome with nothing more than your own good judgment and insight into your loved one's uniqueness. Once you pinpoint their needs, you will be surprised at your ability to eliminate facilities and quickly move a couple to the top of your desirable list. Your options may not always be as satisfactory as you would like. Decisions will weigh heavily on your shoulders. Even placement in a good nursing home may leave you wondering if you made the right selection. It helps to remember that there are no perfect nursing homes, but as a consumer you have the option of setting your own priorities.

The BE AWARE and BEWARE sections help with initial questions. EXAMPLES follow.

BE AWARE
- An efficient beginning is the elimination of some facilities. The Internet (Chapter 5) helps you locate and disregard the worst of facilities.
- Even flawed information collected from multiple sources, i.e., TV, printed advertising, billboards, the Internet, when viewed objectively will probably narrow a search to three or four facilities.
- Special care needs of your loved one such as safety for wandering residents, psychiatric care, smoking policies, wound care, rehabilitation, etc., may eliminate other facilities.
- Those living in smaller communities have the added advantage of talking with medical personnel, friends, neighbors and acquaintances having personal knowledge of nearby facilities. Nurses working in the area have valuable insight; are the residents they encounter from a specific nursing home clean and well nourished?
- Some facilities may be full and simply have a waiting list.
- Expect the first question when you contact a facility to be about your payment source. Your answer determines whether the spokesperson acknowledges the availability of a bed. Chapter 4 is a quick reference.
- After a hospitalization, it is important to consider whether you anticipate a short stay for rehabilitation and a return home, or a permanent move to nursing home care. The determination allows you to use your Medicare payment wisely. Chapter 4 explains Medicare's value.
- A plain vanilla building does not indicate plain vanilla nurses or plain vanilla care. It may be your best option. Plain vanilla can mean profits are funneled into patient care needs instead of

capital improvements meant to increase the building's real estate value.
- The facility sporting manicured lawns, landscaping and impressive facades may spend nothing on inside maintenance such as plumbing, air conditioning, heating, and electrical systems. An on-site visit will help answer these questions (Chapter 6).
- A new nursing home building always presents a challenge to nearby facilities. Families are tempted to choose or relocate their loved ones to the fresh surroundings. The spanking new environment does not necessarily come with better care.

BEWARE
- Many residents come to the nursing home for rehabilitation with the expectation of returning home, but more often become permanent residents.
- Ownership matters, but may be impossible to pinpoint. You cannot depend on not-for-profits, religious and veterans' affiliations to provide any better care than their competitors. Individual facility operations and personnel play a far greater role in good resident care.
- Banners and signs adorning the premises are meaningless: "Facility of the Year," "Top Rated," "Loving Care," " Devoted," etc. The displays are trumped up by corporate marketing departments and rotated between their buildings. If they were accurate, the nursing home would have a waiting list and no need for the bawdy advertising.
- Choices are limited in rural areas. Potential residents often prefer to stay close to home and friends even if the only available facility has a reputation for poor care. If such a choice is made and there are no nearby relatives, frequent visits by a devotee are important in order to recognize problems early on.
- The Center for Medicare and Medicaid (CMS) notes, "Visits by family members can improve both the residents' quality of life and quality of care, it may often be better to select a nursing home that is very close over one that may be, compared to a higher rated nursing home that would be far away." (sic)
- It is very disheartening to be settled into a good nursing home and see care deteriorate, usually after changes in management.

Now you face a decision of whether to stay and advocate for your resident or search for another facility. It is even more discouraging to realize the instability will probably be repeated in a different facility. However, you learned much from your first search which makes the decision to stay or search for another nursing home easier.

EXAMPLE: In this instance a facility is spending resources on landscaping to enhance their façade while ignoring needed maintenance inside the building.

"Miss Frances, can you tell me why they're spending all that money on watering the yard when I still can't get any warm water for my residents?" Gloria, a nurse's aide, referenced the landscaping project on the facility's front lawn. The project's ditches and dirt piles decimated the grass over the lawn's expanse of a quarter city block. New owners were installing an automatic irrigation and sprinkler system.

Inside, one wing of the building had been without hot water for two weeks. Promises of a fix were unfulfilled. Management instructed the nurses' aides to take their residents to another wing of the building for showers. Another nurse's aide said, "Well, it's a lot more work to roll residents over there. The residents don't like it. The halls are cold and there's always a long wait for a shower to open up. After a few showers we always run out of hot water—there's too much strain on the water heaters."

A young nurse's aide added, "I can't stand washing my residents' faces and cleaning their bottoms with cold water. I soak up a batch of washcloths and heat 'em up in the microwave."

I had no answers for the weekend, but left a message for management. The response, "They can just quit complaining and get their residents to a shower that has hot water."

The sprinkler system was completed within two weeks and new sod was in place. Impressive shrubs and oriental grasses added detail. Colorful blooms bordered the long winding sidewalk stretching from the parking lot to the front door. Inside, nurses' aides were still without the hot water they needed to care for sixty residents. Gloria said, "Miss Frances, it's getting worse. Now we don't have enough washcloths. They said there are problems in the laundry so we're just using towels for washcloths. I guess we'll run out of towels pretty soon. If the laundry can't get out washcloths, how can they get out towels?"

After three more weeks and a state inspector's visit, hot water was available and the laundry operated as normal. A few months later, during the summer heat, the new lawn and landscaping were dry and wilting, the flowers were dead. Gloria asked, "Miss Frances, did you see the front yard?"

"Yeah, I did. It needs water."

"Well, there won't be any watering. Seems like they didn't pay the contractor so he came and disconnected the whole thing." None of the new sod or shrubs survived until the next rain. The facility's front acreage was left with nothing more than a couple of ornamental grass clumps.

EXAMPLE: This situation shows that even professionals may have a the tendency to place more importance on a building's age or structural appearance than the care provided by staff.

While working as a wound consultant I received a call from a social worker at a large metropolitan hospital. She knew me as a resource for pressure ulcers and bedsores throughout the area's nursing homes. One of her hospital patients needed nursing home care for extensive bedsores. She asked for a recommendation.

I suggested a nearby facility. It was known for good overall care and excellent bedsore treatment. The Director of Nursing was a retired Navy nurse. He ran a tight ship. Staffing was adequate and the support needed for wound healing was in place. She could expect her patient's bedsores to heal.

The reply, "Oh, Frances. That building is so plain vanilla."

She referred her patient to another facility . . . a recently constructed building. I wondered if she thought the family might more readily accept transfer to a glossy new nursing home.

References
National Consumer Voice for Long-Term Care
McKnights: https://www.mcknights.com/kimberly-marselas/author/1479/

CHAPTER 4

UNDERSTANDING PAYMENT

Until the need arises, few of us have reason to delve into nursing home payment. Your own knowledge may be limited to friends' accounts of wrestling with their loved ones' nursing home expenses. First exposure to costs is mind-boggling. Terms referring to payment only add to the fog: Medicare, Medicaid, Social Security, private pay, applied income, spend down, insurance. The payment network is not as complicated as it seems. However, fitting your payment methods into the variety of nursing home business models may challenge your patience. Learning the basics of payment will give you confidence and clout as you figure out how to pay for the best nursing home.

Few are able to bear the expense of nursing home care on their own. Monthly cost of a semi-private room begins at around $2700; the national median cost is $6700 and there are no upper limits. A Genworth cost survey for 2015 noted semi-private *daily* rates as high as $1255. In expensive areas a semi-private room can easily exceed $100,000 annually. Private rooms begin at $4000 monthly. Although price varies according to regions of the country, annual rate increases are consistent at 3 to 4 percent nationwide.

No one is protected from a catastrophic accident or health crisis requiring lengthy or even permanent nursing home care. It is sobering to realize that even the young may fall into this category, yet health insurance does not pay for extended periods of nursing home care. Today, public funds are also limited, leaving most of us to cobble together payment from a combination of personal and government sources. Personal funds usually include Social Security checks, retirement accounts, pensions and savings accounts. Government programs linked to nursing home payment are Medicare, Medicaid and rarely the Veterans Administration.

Private insurance policies for long-term care flourished for a while, but over time issues with reliability and premium increases have diminished their numbers. The Affordable Care Act originally contained a provision to begin a national long-term care insurance plan with voluntary participation during working years. Congress repealed the Community Living Assistance Services and Supports Act (CLASS) in 2013.

Medicare and Medicaid are often mixed up and used interchangeably during conversations, but they are significantly different programs. You will often hear nursing home staff refer to them as "care" and "caid."

Medicare is *federally* funded health insurance provided to Social Security beneficiaries. Nursing home payment is tied to an illness serious enough to require at least a *three-midnight* hospital admission. Medicare pays the nursing home for continued treatment of that same illness with rehabilitation, therapy and skilled nursing care. A Medicare beneficiary must access this funding within thirty days of the hospital discharge date. The maximum benefit is 100 days and there are many nuances attached. **Think of Medicare as paying for specific therapy and care for a limited time.**

Medicaid in the nursing home is a combination of *federal* and *state* funds paying for care of chronic conditions necessitating twenty-four-hour help because of physical and mental impairments. Most of these residents will require the nursing home's oversight and assistance for the remainder of their lives. Receiving Medicaid benefits is dependent upon financial need. Most residents eventually need Medicaid assistance because their other sources of payment become exhausted. **Think of Medicaid as paying for routine nursing home care over the long haul.**

The other side of payment is what a facility will accept. You may need a strong dose of patience to work through facility references to "financials"—nursing home speak for your method of payment. Government, church and community owned facilities are more flexible in the type of payment they accept. However, their numbers dwindled in recent years and only a few remain. The majority of nursing homes are private enterprises, thus free to decide what kind of payment they accept.

The BE AWARE and BEWARE sections will give insight into understanding why a nursing home may be enthusiastic or uninterested in your inquiry. An EXAMPLE follows.

BE AWARE
- A resident may move through several methods of payment during their need for nursing home care.

- Whether a resident enters a nursing home after a hospitalization or directly from the community greatly impacts early payments and admission possibilities.
- Changing a payment source sometimes means a disruptive move to another facility.

Private pay: All facilities welcome private-pay patients (those able to pay the monthly charges from personal resources).
1. The facility's monthly payment for routine care arrives easily without government paperwork and deadlines.
2. Private payment sometimes provides an opportunity to negotiate monthly rates in facilities accepting multiple payment sources.
3. Some facilities accept only private payment.
4. Most private-pay-only facilities are Medicare certified allowing the nursing home and its residents to capture the financial benefits of Medicare participation. If a private-pay-only nursing home does not participate in the Medicare program their residents must access the Medicare payment in another facility.
5. A resident in a facility accepting only Medicare and private pay will be required to find another facility when Medicare benefits end and they can no longer pay from personal funds.

Medicare Part A: Facilities compete for Medicare Part A (traditional Medicare) patients.
1. Medicare pays nursing homes (skilled nursing facilities) high dollars for skilled care and therapy following a *three-midnight* hospital admission; meaning, the patient occupied a hospital *admission* bed at twelve midnight for three consecutive nights. Hospital stays charged as *observation* are different and do not qualify for admission. See Chapter 7.
2. Medicare provides the patient further treatment and rehabilitation in the nursing home after the hospital admission. The hospital treats the patient's initial symptoms and the nursing home continues skilled nursing treatment and therapy for the same illness.

3. Your share of payment for a Medicare skilled nursing home admission: days 1-20 = $0; days 21-100 = $167.50 per day in 2018; day 101 and beyond, all costs are yours.
4. Some Medicare patients enter the nursing home for therapy and skilled care then return home after rehabilitation. However, most settle into the nursing home with other payment sources.
5. Do not expect to receive 100 days of Medicare benefits. A full 100 days under Medicare is rare. This is not Medicare rationing, rather the facility taking Medicare's top cream and leaving the resident stranded. You see,
    a. The first twenty days of Medicare payment is easy revenue for facilities because Medicare rarely requests clinical records to support the facility charges. The program understands the need for rebuilding strength and reconditioning after being hospitalized.
    b. Beyond 20 days Medicare's payment scrutiny increases, thus few facilities are willing to devote the employee time and resources required to support continued Medicare payment. Without acceptable documentation, the facility faces the risk of denied payment.
    c. Days 21-100 focus on what is reasonable and necessary and very dependent upon a facility's willingness to document and advocate for the benefits.
    d. Such continued payment requires nursing assessment and documentation skills. Short staffing and lack of training contributes to the problem.
    e. Most facilities are satisfied to skim the first 20 low risk payment days and shift further payment responsibility to the resident.
6. Medicare patients can refuse to be removed from Medicare and appeal the facility decision to stop Medicare services. Winning such an appeal is difficult because Medicare's decision is based on facility records,

which rarely reflect the resident's actual medical condition.

Medicare Advantage Part C: Medicare Advantage plans are sold as a replacement for traditional Medicare.
1. Part C plans limit skilled nursing facility choices and care through restricted networks, contractual agreements and case manager decisions.
2. These limitations and slow payment leave few facilities willing to accept residents with Advantage plans.

Medicaid: A majority of nursing homes accept Medicaid payment.
1. Medicaid accounts for the largest number of nursing home residents across the country. According to the Center for Disease Control, the national average for combined partial and total Medicaid payment is 63 percent of nursing home residents.
2. In order to receive Medicaid benefits in a nursing home, a resident must first meet a financial need, then establish the need for twenty-four-hour care and oversight.
3. Establishing financial eligibility varies by state but a few general rules apply.
    a. Approval is based on limited property and assets.
    b. A resident is usually allowed to disregard a home, car and around two thousand dollars in additional assets.
    c. Burial policies are not considered an asset.
    d. Spousal protections make sure a spouse retains the resources needed to continue living independently in the community while a husband or wife receives nursing home benefits.
    e. Financial applications are the resident or responsible party's task and usually involve collecting information for a look back period from the previous five years.
    f. Residents must "spend down" resources to the two thousand dollar asset limit in order to reach Medicaid eligibility. The process usually involves

the sale of property and assets with the proceeds used to pay for the resident's care until the two thousand dollar asset limit is reached.
4. Establishing the need for twenty-four-hour care and oversight is the nursing home's responsibility.
5. Once again, state guidelines vary, but the standard is generally based on a resident's need for help with bathing, dressing, feeding, toileting, medications and safety.
   a. The nursing home's assessment of the resident's limitations and needs determines whether the resident will receive Medicaid payment assistance. This assessment also establishes the daily payment rate or level of care.
   b. The amount Medicaid pays a facility is based on the complexity of care and the amount of time employees spend caring for the patient and is called the *level of care*.
   c. Some facilities may not be interested in pursuing the initial application if they foresee a basic or low level of care, which they interpret as a low daily payment rate.
   d. The same facility might view a more complex Medicaid patient as worth their time in the evaluation and application process. Because the resident's needs are greater, the level of care and the daily payment rate increases.
6. Medicaid pays 100 percent of only a few residents' nursing home costs. The more likely picture is a resident's monthly fixed income paying a portion of the monthly charge and Medicaid paying the remainder.
7. Most residents' monthly income consists of Social Security and pension checks. They are applied to the nursing home's charges and aptly called *applied income*. Medicaid pays the balance of the monthly rate. For example, a resident receiving $1400 Social Security monthly plus a state retiree pension of $900 has a total applied income of $2300. The nursing home charge is $4000 leaving $1700 for Medicaid to pay.

Long Term Care Insurance: Few policies approach the full cost of nursing home care.
1. Most nursing homes will not assume the responsibility for monthly billing to an insurance company.
2. Monthly payments are usually issued to the resident or responsible party.
3. The funds are figured into a resident's applied income if Medicaid application is necessary.

Veterans: Possibilities for the Veterans Administration (VA) paying for nursing home care are quite limited even though nursing home marketing may tout VA connections.
1. There is a difference between a facility focusing on veterans' care and Veterans Administration (VA) payment for care in any facility.
2. Any VA payment possibility begins by establishing eligibility within the VA system.
3. The VA contracts with a few nursing homes in each state to provide care at the VA's expense. The veteran becomes a regular nursing home resident, but the payment is often limited to a few months.
4. Community Living Centers (VA Nursing Homes) are usually located within or near VA complexes and are owned and controlled by the VA. Residency in the VA's Community Living Centers is funded by the VA. Formerly known as VA Nursing Homes, they offer specialized care in some instances, but mostly focus on creating a community and "home" atmosphere. The number of rooms provided through this program is limited and vacancies are few. Obtaining the care is usually dependent upon an advocate within the VA system and surviving a waiting list.
5. State Veterans Homes have no association with the VA other than the veterans who are residents there. State veterans homes were conceived after the Civil War to house needy veterans. They are still owned by state governments, but the operation in most states is contracted out to nursing home management companies. Even though admission is limited to veterans and their

families, the facility is operated just like any other nursing home. Payment comes from the same sources as other nursing homes in the community: private pay, Medicare, Medicaid, long-term care insurance.

BEWARE
- The quality of resident care cannot vary according to payment source. States issue each nursing home a license to operate based on providing each resident within that facility the same competent care.
- Expect the first question on your initial contact to be your payment source. The spokesperson's response usually depends on how you will pay.
- It is helpful to realize that most nursing homes are private businesses even though corporately owned. If you cannot pay the asking price for their product (nursing home care), they are under no obligation to provide you the product. If a method of payment does not fit their business model an inquiry may be rejected.
- Nursing homes are masters at adhering to all state and federal laws against discrimination while simultaneously discriminating against some admissions. For example: a private pay facility rejecting a resident whose funds are limited and will soon be dependent upon Medicaid funding, a potential resident who is perceived to have behavior problems, a resident requiring time consuming or expensive physical care, treatments and equipment or racial and gender preferences.
- There is no limit to the amount a facility can charge a private pay resident for the same care all other residents receive.
- Use Medicare days wisely. They can become a bargaining chip for a desired nursing home. Facilities are more receptive to accepting patients with low daily Medi*caid* payment rates when they can capture the resident's high Medi*care* payments up front. For instance, a hospitalized patient may be discharged to different settings, which bill Medi*care* for skilled nursing care, i.e. their 100 days of Medicare. Examples are: hospitals direct patients to their skilled nursing unit, private pay nursing homes may keep them only as long as their Medicare days last, or rural hospitals' swing beds; all of which bill against the precious 100

days of Medicare billing. If the desired facility is left with only a few or perhaps no Medicare days they may not look as favorably on a Medi*caid* resident.
- Medicare participation allows facilities to capture daily reimbursement rates much higher than regular payment sources. An additional financial advantage is shifting the building's operating expenses to a federal program through an annual cost report.
- During the first twenty days of a Medicare stay all the resident's private sources of nursing home payment stop. The resident retains their Social Security, pension checks and all their applied income. For Medicare days twenty-one to one hundred the resident retains all their income except the coinsurance of $167.50 in 2018 (future years' costs are undecided at print time). Medicaid pays the coinsurance for the few residents receiving 100 percent of their nursing home care through Medicaid.
- While a resident is receiving Medicare skilled care, the nursing home is responsible for the Medicare billing. The resident is only expected to pay the nursing home the coinsurance for days 21-100. A facility cannot bill a Medicare resident for charges Medicare did not pay. The nursing home has the option of appealing denied payment by proving the care was reasonable and necessary.
- Medicare pays for complex nursing procedures such as wound care, intravenous therapy and nutritional support throughout the 100 days if the treatment is daily.
- The Medicare program is specific in its obligation to provide reasonable and necessary care after an illness. The goal is always to return the resident to their pre-illness activity level. If a patient was walking before a hospitalization and can no longer stand up, it is reasonable to give the resident a chance to walk again. Sometimes a catastrophic illness such as a stroke makes it impossible for the same patient to walk again. Still, during the recovery period, every Medicare recipient deserves a chance to reach his/her maximum ability—maybe walking with a cane, using a walker or wheelchair.
- There has been a common message when stopping therapy on Medicare patients: "The patient has reached a *plateau*." In rehab

jargon, plateau means the resident is not showing improvement. The reference is to a progress graph showing an upward trend, similar to a mountain, before reaching a horizontal line resembling a flat plateau. Don't be surprised if your resident reaches their plateau near the twentieth Medicare day and you are told, "Medicare won't pay for their *maintenance.*" However, this message is changing.

Maintenance is the upkeep of exercises and therapeutic activities needed to prevent a resident from losing ground after rehabilitation. In the example above, if a resident is walking with a cane at the end of his Medicare nursing home therapy (the plateau) he will probably need exercises and an activity regimen in order to sustain his ability to walk with a cane. Usually, a resident is referred to the nursing home's restorative program for an exercise plan carried out by a certified nursing assistant. The program can be adequate, but it is rarely staffed sufficiently to provide the time and attention residents need.

A recent federal court decision, *Jimmo v. Sebelius,* overturned the previous mindset that Medicare does not pay for maintenance. Facilities and providers are transitioning to the new rules; Medicare pays for maintenance as long as skilled care is required. For example, a resident plateaus for physical therapy twenty days after admission, but continues to receive Medicare skilled nursing home care for other problems; the resident can now receive maintenance physical therapy for the additional skilled care period. During the transition some health care providers may operate under the old misconception and deny maintenance care for physical, occupational and speech therapy.

- In some facilities, the mix of resident payment sources and amounts factor into administrators' and nursing directors' bonus packages. Their bonus goals are tied to attaining the budget's projected room rate mix. A realistic budget usually includes a couple of private pay residents, around fifteen percent Medicare patients and the remainder Medicaid. However, Medicaid does not pay the same for each resident, rather graduated amounts based on the level of care needed. A typical facility budget allows a few token Medicaid residents with low payment rates and sets higher occupancy numbers for

the medium to high paying levels of care. Even residents paying most of their costs with applied income and needing only a few monthly dollars from Medicaid fall into this plan. Therefore, admission may rest more on payment source than availability.
- As a consumer you have your own leverage. Profitability depends upon keeping the building occupied. Most admissions gain favor when an administrator faces the probability of empty beds for more than a few days.
- For Medicaid residents, their level of care payment determines the maximum amount a facility can charge for their nursing home care.
- Once Medicaid's initial assessment for care and payment is completed, the information follows the resident. In a move to another facility the level of care is transferred and payment continues at the same level.
- A Medicaid resident contributing some applied income (personal funds) to their nursing home cost is allowed to keep a personal needs allowance of $30 to $60 monthly. If Medicaid pays the total nursing home cost, the resident usually receives no personal allowance. The amount varies by state.
- Even though a veteran, every resident of the State Veterans Home faces the same payment structures as described above. It is helpful to remember that corporate management companies operate these facilities the same as all other nursing homes.

EXAMPLE: How a Medicaid resident's inquiry was first rejected, but later welcomed.

My sister Jean was on the phone, "I think Mother's ready for a nursing home and pretty soon. She's needing more help and now she won't eat." For years Jean and her husband, Dick, managed Mother's care in assisted living facilities. We shared a longstanding agreement; They would manage her assisted living care and I would take responsibility when nursing home care became necessary.

Mother's Social Security and her state employee pension were sufficient to pay for assisted living, but fell short of the monthly cost for nursing home care. She had no assets and needed Medicaid assistance for the remainder. The necessity of twenty-four-hour care seemed evident; she needed help bathing, dressing, and taking medications. Mother was confused, needed assistance to manage severe joint pain and protection from recurring falls. Lung disease required oxygen at times.

My brother-in-law filed the application for Medicaid financial eligibility while I began searching for a nursing home. My first stop was our local facility. Ann, the Director of Nursing, showed no interest in my inquiry.

She said, "I don't think your mother will qualify for Medicaid."

I knew Mother met Medicaid requirements, but the decision was Ann's. I also understood the reason for Ann's rejection. This rural nursing home did not have another facility within twenty miles. She had no interest in spending the time and effort required to complete a Medicaid assessment and application. In the absence of a competing facility, the community furnished her with a continual source of referrals and payment choices.

Work around San Antonio led me to a small nursing home. The Director of Nursing, Laurie, was young, innovative, energetic, and totally involved in her residents' care. She assured me, "Your mother will certainly qualify for Medicaid."

Undaunted by the assessment and eligibility paperwork, she accepted Mother as a resident. We paid her Social Security and pension benefits to the nursing home. When Medicaid benefits were approved, the program paid their portion retroactively to her admission date.

The San Antonio nursing home worked well until Laurie resigned. Soon afterward, a shipwreck ensued within the facility. I had to find a better place for Mother and inquired at the local nursing home again. It seemed like a logical move since it was only five minutes from my home, I could visit her daily.

Now that her "financials" were established with a high Medicaid payment rate and substantial applied income she seemed like a more desirable admission. Over the next few weeks, I received several calls from Ann's admissions coordinator promoting the benefits of "our home." Mother's financials moved seamlessly with her from the San Antonio nursing home to the local facility.

References

"The Challenge of Financing Long-Term Care," Judy Feder, Ph.D., Saint Louis University School of Law. On URBAN institute website.

ADVANTAGE MEDICARE: Congress approved the creation of Advantage Medicare C plans in the 1990s with the insurance industry's promise of better care for decreased cost. The plans support healthy lifestyles and cut medical care through cost-conscious networks of doctors and hospitals, i.e. limited choices for their enrollees. Most participants are satisfied with the care until they face declining health or a catastrophic illness. In July 2017 Kaiser Health News (KHN) called attention to a Government Accounting Office (GAO) report adding weight to criticisms that some Medicare Advantage health plans may leave sicker patients worse off. The KHN title: "As Seniors Get Sicker, They're More Likely to Drop Medicare Advantage Plans."

SWING BED: The term Medicare uses to describe a hospital room that can switch from acute care (hospital) status to skilled care (nursing home). Charges for a stay in a swing bed are billed as Medicare skilled nursing facility care and therefore are a part of the 100 days allotted for skilled nursing facility care. Medicare days spent in a hospital swing bed are no longer available in the nursing home. The hospitals typically use most of the twenty days that Medicare pays at 100 percent and then seek nursing home placement.

QUALIFYING FOR PAYMENT

Medicare: https://www.medicare.gov/coverage/skilled-nursing-facility-care.html

Medicaid: https://www.medicaid.gov/medicaid/ltss/index.html

Veterans Administration: http://www.va.gov/GERIATRICS/Guide/LongTermCare/VA_Community_Living_Centers.asp#

OVERVIEW OF COSTS
https://www.genworth.com/dam/Americas/US/PDFs/Consumer/corporate/130568_040115_gnw.pdf

Jimmo V. Sebelius Corrective Action Plan for people living with MS, Parkinson's, Alzheimer's, paralysis and other long-term conditions: www.cms.gov/Center/Special-Topic/Jimmo-Center.

CHAPTER 5

INTERNET RESOURCES

A good place to begin your pursuit of a good nursing home is the Internet. Much of the information found there is wide-ranging and generic. It comes from multiple sources including advocacy groups, elder organizations, the media and industry trade groups, to name a few. Except for news reports of individual facility incidents, the material is usually nonspecific, useful for overall insight, but short on the statistics needed to compare one facility to another.

Efficient side-by-side comparisons become important when faced with an urgent need and short time frame. Where to start? You may know of a nearby nursing home. A hospital social worker might recommend a skilled nursing facility. You can Google nursing homes in your area code. Select several for your research, always remembering that different labels are only marketing tools. Care centers, nursing and rehabilitation centers and skilled nursing facilities are all nursing homes.

Internet resources are helpful in narrowing choices and saving time, but the information gleaned is only the beginning. I suggest a three-pronged internet approach: (1) facility websites (2) Center for Medicare and Medicaid (CMS) star rating system (3) CMS inspection reports.

First, check each facility's website, but consider these sites reliable for only three bits of information:
- What kind of payment they accept (this may allow you to eliminate some facilities immediately)
- Total number of resident beds in the building (large facilities generally have more layers of management making problem-solving more difficult)
- Claims of specialized care such as wounds, bedsores and dementia (helpful if your loved one needs such care).

Expect enhanced photos of the building and landscaping because marketing focuses on the facility's physical setting. Declarations of caring, loving, dedicated, devoted, top-ranked, number one, etc. appeal to our emotions but are also advertised by facilities with the worst of care.

Second, go to Nursing Home Compare, the Center for Medicare and Medicaid Services (CMS) website: medicare.gov/nursinghomecompare. From here you can begin side-by-side facility comparisons. CMS condenses information about *inspection*s, *staffing*, and *quality measures* into a rating system of one to five stars. Additionally, using information collected for these three areas, CMS determines an *overall* star rating. Five stars represent the best quality, designated as *Much Above Average*. Advocates recommend avoiding a facility with one star considered *Much Below Average* or two stars, *Below Average*.

Third, I suggest drilling further into the CMS website to: data.medicare.gov/Nursing-Home-Compare/Deficiencies. Here a spreadsheet reveals a history of facility deficiencies and type, whether found on a survey (annual inspection) or complaint investigation. The term "deficiency" indicates failure to meet *minimum* standards. I do not trust facilities with lists of deficiencies year after year, especially the same deficiencies.

I hope you will think of these websites as a guide, routing you toward a good nursing home, by avoiding bad ones. Facilities "game" the inspection and reporting system. Numbers may be outdated and changes in ownership skew the data. Even with shortcomings the CMS site still offers the best starting point for facility comparison.

The BE AWARE and BEWARE sections offer condensed information and EXAMPLES follow. APPENDIX A offers a deeper dive into the Star rating system and its history.

BE AWARE
- Individual facility websites will not give a hint of any shortcomings whatsoever.
- At <medicare.gov/nursinghomecompare> you can review facility inspections, correction dates, star ratings, fines and penalties. Using percentages the site also compares the facility to state and national averages.
- Ratings matter over the long haul. A nursing home may seem okay until an injury occurs. It is far better to be in a higher rated facility when something goes wrong.

- If a nursing home has no deficiencies, it means that it met *minimum* standards at the time of inspection. Inspections do not identify nursing homes that give outstanding care.
- CMS cautions that their Five-Star rating system has strengths and limitations.
- The goals of CMS star ratings are two-fold: First, to help consumers make distinctions between high and low performing nursing homes; second, to help nursing homes identify areas needing improvement.
- The *Year 5 Report* (2014) suggested improved performance since the Star ratings began in 2008, but found it impossible to determine whether improvements reflect changes in reporting or changes in practice. The public is left to ask, "Has care really improved or have facilities gamed the reporting process?"
- *Abt Associates Inc.* who conducted the *Year 5 Report* observed that changes in *quality measures* and *staffing* were based on data self-reported by the nursing homes. Resident advocates questioned these self-reporting portions. In 2017 CMS began collecting staffing numbers from electronic payroll records and a few of the quality measures are ranked from facility billing submitted to Medicare and Medicaid. These claims are subject to audit for accuracy and are therefore more reliable. Some of the data in the quality measures remains dependent upon the reliability of the facility and honesty of the employee completing the data entry.
- Quality measures attempt to compare the worth of care provided by each facility. Data collection originates within a standard resident assessment (Minimum Data Set or MDS) form, which is submitted electronically. My experience is that accuracy depends upon the skill and integrity of employees.
- An improvement made during 2016 was the Five-Star comparison for short-stay or rehabilitation residents. The short-stay rating system is intended to give consumers an opportunity to compare statistics for those patients admitted after a hospitalization for therapy and skilled care. Specifically, did the patient recover and return home or become a long-term resident of the facility after 100 days. Medicare Advantage Plans are not included in the short-stay data.

- It is difficult to compare facilities located in different states. Even though the standards are the same across the country, there are variations in how different states carry out the inspection process.
- There is a link to the state agency website at the end of each facility's review on <medicare.gov/nursinghomecompare>.
- A few facilities (private pay) do not participate in the Medicare or Medicaid program. Therefore, their data is absent from the CMS website. These nursing homes are subject to the same state health and safety inspections as CMS facilities. Their data is available from their state regulatory agency and a link is available at <medicare.gov/nursinghomecompare>.
- CMS intends that the Five Star nursing home ratings be used with other sources of information and cannot substitute for visiting the nursing home.

BEWARE
- The quality of a nursing home may get much better or much worse in a short period of time. Improvement and decline usually involve cycles of increased staffing, stocking supplies, updating documentation, and maintenance repairs in preparation for an anticipated inspection or after a bad inspection. When the inspection is completed and deficiencies are corrected, most facilities cut staff and return to their same old practices.
- Bankruptcies and sales often occur when deficiencies and fines become very expensive for profiteers to resolve. Many layers of corporate ownership shield the responsibility and identity of these unscrupulous practitioners even though they continue circulating from the old organization to a new one and from one facility to another.
- Sale of a nursing home deletes the nursing home's history from the CMS website and the data begins anew with only an initial inspection recorded. Years of negligent care within a building are erased from consumers' sight even though the prospects for improvement are slim.
- Only eleven of eighteen possible quality measures are used when determining star ratings. Among those *not* in the mix are

incontinence, mental and social functioning, feeding tubes, nutrition, medication errors and unnecessary drugs.
- Nursing homes are experts at gaming the *inspections* component of the five star ratings. They do so by creating a false picture of the care being provided during the few days inspectors are present in the building. The most widespread tactic is having additional staff on hand, actually enough to care for residents. Intense prior preparation with corporate swat teams and mock inspections also influences inspection outcomes. More details are available in Appendix A.
- Untold dollars are invested in the purchase of computer programs designed to capture resident needs, generate care plans, document care, transmit to regulatory agencies and send payment claims to Medicare and Medicaid. The prevailing question is always whether residents receive the care. Problems often begin with nurses' aides' erroneous or absent bedside documentation; licensed professionals add to the inaccuracies, or the data entry person may simply click through program prompts without verifying that care was provided.

EXAMPLE: This shows the importance of staffing and taking an objective view of the overall ratings when using the CMS star system.

A Center for Medicare and Medicaid Services (CMS) tip: Quality is generally better in nursing homes that have more staff working directly with residents.

I recently logged onto <medicare.gov/nursinghomecompare>. A review of five-star ratings in my area found a facility with *one star* for staffing (much below average) and *five stars* for quality measures (much above average). How could that be? My conclusion: The facility is very good at gaming the quality measures. It is impossible to provide five star care with one star staffing.

Another facility had *one* star ratings for staffing, quality measures and overall. Their inspection rated *two* stars with many deficiencies and several complaints recorded. I looked further into their survey history at <data.medicare.gov/Nursing-Home-Compare/Deficiencies/>. Facility histories go back three years. This nursing home has pages of recorded deficiencies and complaint investigations throughout that time, yet there have been no fines, penalties or payment denials.

Rather than waste time with analysis, it seems reasonable to follow advocates advice and avoid nursing homes with one or two stars whenever possible.

EXAMPLE: A national chain's pattern of dangerous care leading to crisis, corrections and then a return to the same predictable cycle of poor care.

According to my new employer, "Everything that could go wrong did go wrong during our inspection." I was the new Director of Nursing for a facility facing fines and threats of closure if dangerous health deficiencies weren't corrected within seven days. Lesser problems would take months to resolve. The survey results comprised a thick volume of deficiencies—the most I had seen in fifteen years of nursing home experience.

The salary was hard to resist. The regional manager promised both myself, and the young new administrator all the resources and support we needed. As is usually the case following catastrophic inspections, the previous administrator and director of nurses had been fired. The facility was being managed by regional personnel, anxious to pass the responsibility on to someone else.

We dug in with long hours on the job. The 220-bed facility was woefully understaffed so we set about hiring new employees and implementing corrections. Two additional registered nurses rounded out the new staff. After six months, the deficiencies were corrected and the facility was almost at capacity with 218 residents. The administrator reported profits. Much of the stress was behind us.

Within a month the corporation's regional office directed us to cut staffing hours. As Director of Nursing I was purposefully slow in doing so because less staff would mean deteriorating resident care. The corporation hired a staffing coordinator to control the nursing department's schedule and implement the changes.

As nursing assistant hours dwindled so did the attention residents received. Disappointed in their ability to care for residents, both registered nurses resigned within a few months. After facing the reality that my presence only perpetuated the bad situation, I resigned also.

Like many Directors of Nursing, such circumstances occur more than once in our careers. This was just the most physically and emotionally draining for me. The residents and families who had become accustomed to personal attention and treatment were returning to the same substandard care identified on the inspection—not because I was leaving, but because of dangerous staffing levels.

EXAMPLE: How the star rating system can be used for comparison with a facility's local image, and highlights the problem of finding a good nursing home in rural areas.

In a 2015 article, Kaiser Health News reported *A Top-Rated Nursing Home is Hard to Find in Texas, 10 Other States*. The analysis by the Kaiser Family Foundation found that Texas has the highest percentage of one and two-star homes in the country: 51 percent of its nursing homes are rated "below average," or "much below average," on Nursing Home Compare.

Louisiana is close behind at 49 percent, with Oklahoma, Georgia and West Virginia tying for third at 46 percent. The article continues, "states with at least 40 percent of homes ranked at the bottom two rungs include North Carolina, Tennessee, Kentucky, Ohio, Pennsylvania and New York."

The article gives the example of a family in Lockhart, Texas. Their mother was in a local nursing home because they knew frequent visits are beneficial. The facility seemed pleasant and colorful. Awards from a local newspaper survey proclaimed it the "Best Nursing Home in Caldwell County."

The family's complaints about a windowsill needing repair were ignored. One night, their mother was attacked by fire ants injecting venom into her face, arms, hands and chest. She never recovered and died a few months later. The family's complaint to the Texas regulatory agency was answered with a determination that there was not enough evidence and the windowsill had been fixed.

This family was unaware of the facility's CMS star rating of one star for staffing and quality measures. Had they checked the CMS ratings they would have found nine of ten nursing homes within a twenty-five mile radius got only one or two stars. Only one nursing home, about 20 miles away, earned four or five stars.

References

In a *New York Times* article, "Medicare Star Ratings Allow Nursing Homes to Game the System," Katie Thomas details how nursing homes have learned to game the star rating system to "seriously mislead consumers, and others about conditions at the homes." https://nyti.ms/1mFUPhZ

The five-year report (2014) was conducted by Abt Associates, Inc. and is available at www.cms.gov/Medicare/Provider-Enrollment-and-Certification and Compliance/Downloads/NHC-Year-Five-Report.pdf

http://khn.org/news/a-top-rated-nursing-home-is-hard-to-find-in-texas-10-other-states/

http://www.dispatch.com/content/stories/local/2015/05/14/ohio-fares-poorly-in-nursing-home-study.html

http://www.nytimes.com/2015/02/21/business/nursing-home-ratings-fall-as-tougher-standards-take-effect.html?_r=0

http://khn.org/morning-breakout/nursing-home-quality-scores-drop-after-new-rating-system/

CHAPTER 6

VISIT

Nursing home visits are enlightening. Walking through facilities offers the opportunity to apply your own good sense to the never-ending claims of *quality care*. We hear of *quality of life* and *individualized care* ad nauseam, yet the general perception of nursing homes remains—bad odors and hallways lined with drooling residents asleep in wheelchairs. Expect more. Odors happen occasionally, but should not meet you at the front door. Rows of residents parked in hallways is mostly a situation of the past.

Every nursing home has its own personality. No facility is perfect, and negatives will surface soon enough. Differences in focus and care become evident as you visit in a variety of buildings. I encourage you to put aside preconceived beliefs of nursing home care, whether expecting low performance or unrealistic thoughts of high performance. If you begin visits with an idea of what you seek for your loved one, it will be easier to judge the offerings of each facility.

Much is written about prodding questions to ask the staff on your visit: "Do you like your job? Would you bring your mother here?" Expecting employees' answers to be helpful in the presence of the administrative person guiding you around the building is not realistic, nor will you be given the privacy needed for honest answers.

I suggest you look for competence, comfort and cleanliness during your walk through the building. What you see may be more significant than the guide's selective message or personal questions directed to the staff. Your observations can spur confidence or questions of how your loved one might adjust to this nursing home.

Competence of individual staff members is hard for a visitor to pinpoint. However, whether the facility at large is competent in caring for residents will be obvious. Understaffing, poor supervision and organization will be evidenced by nursing assistants rushing about, nurses oblivious to your unfamiliar face, failure of staff to greet you, an uncomfortable noise level, call lights buzzing and a lack of enthusiasm by your guide. Vacant rooms and beds could be an indication of poor care.

As a visitor you are quite capable of judging comfort, both physical and mental. Happy residents and employees are the benchmark of comfort. Stressed employees may be unable to attend to residents' wellbeing and provide even small comforts. Are restraints being used instead of personal attention? I would consider residents awkwardly positioned in recliners, slipping out of wheelchairs or repetitively seeking help to be uncomfortable. Happy residents and employees are a benchmark of comfort.

Cleanliness goes beyond the polished floors of the reception area and hallways. Indeed, if they are not waxed and polished you have observed your first negative. Most facilities strive to make your first impression a good one. Are baseboards, wheelchair armrests and wheels, air vents and utility carts clean? Take into account odors and unkempt residents wearing stained, dirty clothing.

Someone in the facility should have answers to your concerns about how they will attend to your loved one's idiosyncrasies and specific needs (to the bathroom at midnight, medications at specific times or a firm mattress). The best check on assurances about care is to return unannounced after business hours. Saturday or Sunday afternoons offer an opportunity to talk with visiting families.

Additional insight is presented in the BE AWARE and BEWARE sections and EXAMPLES follow. As you add visit observations to your Internet information expect to gain confidence in your ability to identify quality care.

BE AWARE
- Large national chains are more likely to spend money on capital improvements than enough staffing or patient care necessities such as linen, food and equipment. The enhancements are most often the high visibility areas: landscaping, entryways, reception areas, offices, hallways and dining rooms. A better indication of management's mindset is the condition of resident rooms, nurse's stations and laundry.
- Taking a walk-through visit is the best chance to gauge the facility as a whole. Consider residents' moods, staff attention, lively activity, dismal atmosphere, restraints, noise, lighting, overflowing trash cans, etc. The vitality of residents met in

hallways is a good indicator of the staff's individual attention to each.
- Satisfying your loved one's personal preferences will add a great deal to their feeling of security and happiness. Ask if staff will be able to fulfill non-routine requests: a glass of wine at bedtime, prune juice for breakfast, a bird feeder outside their window, etc.
- The nursing home will be determining whether to accept your loved one for admission while you are deciding if you trust the facility with their care. Beyond personal preferences, being specific about their needs will prevent later misunderstandings: incontinent care, needs to be fed, cannot chew, does not understand instructions, belligerent at times, needs help walking, cannot speak English, etc.
- In addition to improving abilities of residents admitted for rehabilitation, the nursing home is expected to maintain any new resident's functional capacity. Asking about their ability to keep your loved one moving, mentally alert, or continent, for example, will give a feel for their priorities. Questions might be: "Mother needs help getting to the bathroom fast, otherwise she loses control of her urine. Can you help with that? Can someone help Dad walk every day?"
- Nurse call systems such as buzzers, bells and lights (signal lights above doors), which stay on over a couple of minutes, probably indicate short staffing. The fewer call signals the more responsive staff has become in anticipating patient needs—probably the result of adequate staffing. If you see or hear nothing from the nurse call system it has probably been muted or turned off completely.
- Inquiry visits will usually be scheduled to avoid mealtimes which are the busiest hours of the day and most likely to reveal short staffing. Even a good dining room may seem chaotic to a visitor. Also, all staff is needed to concentrate on attending to the residents. Even one staff member lost to guiding a visitor interferes with the mealtime routine.
- The food service supervisor is a key staff person. They are responsible for the kitchen and meal preparation. An introduction and the opportunity to ask questions about your loved one's food preferences are helpful.

- Each facility provides a monthly menu. It should be posted in the dining room or you can ask for a copy. Consider how it compares with your person's food likes and dislikes.
- Meals are usually scheduled between 7:00 a.m. and 5:00 p.m. leaving twelve to thirteen hours between dinner and breakfast. The kitchen is closed, but some facilities have a variety of snacks available at the nurses' station; others have none. Snacks and refreshments are part of the food budget, so asking about their availability and variety hints of a generous versus tight food budget.
- The activities (recreation) director is an informative person to meet. They usually know their residents well and are able to make adjustments for individual interests.
- A calendar is prepared for each month's activities and posted throughout the building. The activities director will be glad to give you a copy to compare with your loved one's interest. Look for creative activities such as music, art, opportunities to paint or sew.
- Accommodations can be made for residents unable to attend group activities, i.e., bedside music, audio books and visits to engage in conversation.
- Weekends without activities are dismal. Scheduled diversions, often conducted by volunteers, are helpful.
- Religious participation is a source of wellbeing for many residents and crucial for the devout. If the activity schedule does not reflect spiritual gatherings suitable for your loved one, the activity director will be able to answer your questions and make accommodations.
- Your visit is a good time to ask about personal TV policies. Friction often develops around roommates' programming, hours of use and volume. Competing TVs in a semiprivate room is nerve racking. Some residents find any TV annoying, especially a roommate's TV.
- Most facilities have a community TV room. Consider whether residents sitting there seem interested in the programming or perhaps were placed there for staff's convenience.
- The laundry is important enough to be included on your visit. It plays a significant role in satisfaction and expense if clothing is

lost or damaged. Stacks of dirty laundry do not bode well for efficiency.
- It is reasonable to ask to view the room or a similar room your loved one would occupy. If you encounter hesitancy about seeing a specific room, move to asking about which hallway they would be on. Accommodations may vary from one hallway to another.
- Seeing a resident bathroom on their probable hallway gives significant insight. Cleanliness, odors, leaking faucets, rusty plumbing, water damage, baseboards needing repair, low toilets and the absence of handicap adjustments (faucets, door knobs and pull-up bars) are safety issues (falls and infections).
- Smoking rules, designated areas and times can be a source of agitation for both the smoker and non-smoker. Will the person who smokes accept facility policy? Are non-smokers protected from smoke?

BEWARE
- The facility is required to have a copy of their last inspection available. Be wary of excuses or complaints of an unfair inspection.
- You can have a better grasp of their inspections if you review them online prior to your visit. Then you will have knowledge of their weaknesses and a basis for questions: data.medicare.gov/Nursing-Home-Compare/Deficiencies.
- When you are there at mealtime (probably on your weekend or after hours return visit) see if the meal served follows the menu. Ways to skimp on the budget inlcude substituting cheaper foods and giving smaller servings. This practice is most prevalent at evening meals when there is less chance of oversight.
- Empty chairs in the dining room may mean residents are being served in their rooms because short staffing leaves employees unable to move residents to the dining room.
- Empty chairs in the dining room can also mean the nursing home census is low. Is the facility short on residents because of poor care?
- You will know the facility's resident capacity from your Internet search. I suggest asking "How many residents do you have in

the nursing home *today*?" If you subtract today's occupancy from the capacity and arrive at more than ten percent vacancy, there may be serious problems within the building.
- Most nursing homes have both a *Resident* Council and *Family* Council in place. The Resident Council is mandated by the facility's licensure. Family Council is not a requirement. However, the absence of a Family Council is a red flag, indicating the nursing home's lack of interest in family participation. Theoretically, both groups contribute ideas to improve the facility and resident care. I suggest asking about both groups and how often they meet.

EXAMPLE: A notation that anxious residents and those seeking help are a significant indication of short staffing and poor care on your visit.

"Help me, help me. Mister, please help me," the thin, frail lady pleaded as my son attempted to maneuver around her wheelchair solidly parked in the only entry to the nursing home. He was visiting his grandmother who had been admitted a few hours earlier. He gently greeted the resident as he continued trying to wiggle around the wheelchair.

"Help me, help me. Mister, please help me," the thin, frail lady pleaded.

My son attempted to maneuver around her wheelchair blocking the nursing home entrance. His grandmother had been admitted a few hours earlier. He was visiting her for the first time. He greeted the resident and continued efforts to wiggle around the wheelchair.

"Oh Mister, you've got to help me," she pleaded.

"Of course ma'am, what do you need?"

"I need to know if my car's out there," she replied, then strained to look outside."

"I'm sure your car's out there."

The resident seemed upset, "I'm afraid it's been stolen."

He reassured her again noting he had just come from the parking lot and everything was okay.

The lady was near tears, anxious and begging, "Mister, please, please help me."

With the resident becoming distraught he finally agreed, "Sure ma'am, I'll go check on your car. What kind of a car do you have?"
"It's a green Studebaker," she answered. He chuckled, shook his head, reassured her again and proceeded on his way.
There is much wrong with this scenario. Most importantly, a resident should not endure such painful anxiety, an uninformed consumer left her in the same anxious state or maybe worse than when he found her, where was the nursing staff and what kind of management would allow such a situation from a safety standpoint as well as the negative perception for visitors to the nursing home. Certainly, this lady would have been receiving personal attention if inspectors had been in the building.

EXAMPLE: A friend's experience highlights the importance of addressing personal preferences and habits.

The family patriarch agreed on his move to the nursing home, but was adjusting poorly. The new resident had many complaints, seemed miserable and was not sleeping well. A son remembered his father's longstanding evening toddy and arranged for a shot of whiskey at bedtime. The resident began to sleep well and soon settled into the nursing home routine.

EXAMPLE: How comparison visits to nursing homes can avoid uncertainty after admission.

The young dental hygienist was near tears, "He wants to go home. He needs to take care of his pickup truck and things at the house."
Her father had been in the nursing home less than forty-eight hours. The resident seemed unaware that he was on a secure or locked unit. Unlike most new residents, he was not trying to open

the locked doors and leave, he was just very sad. He was looking to her for help.

His daughter said, "I had to do something. He's been mixed up and the neighbors say he wanders into the street at all hours. I'd like to bring him to my house, but I'm at work all day."

She was considering moving her father to a nearby nursing home with "VA connections." She thought he might be happier there, but she had not visited that facility. During our conversation, the daughter said, "I made financial arrangements and just took a quick look at the room before bringing him here."

I encouraged her to determine what care she expects for her father, then visit different nursing homes; there were several in the area with secure units. Also, after her visits to determine the best facility for her father. I told her, it will take several weeks for him to settle into any new living arrangements. However, the value of careful visits will serve as her satisfaction that Father is in the best nursing home for him. I also informed her the facility she referenced had no VA connections beyond their advertisements.

Father and daughter sat side by side, without talking, for a long time. She left in tears after expressing gratitude for the advice received.

The resident was transferred to another nursing home within a few weeks.

References

CENSUS: Reference to the number of residents in the building.

INSPECTION REPORT:
In a few instances a recent inspection may not have been posted on the nursing home compare website, <medicare.gov/nursing home compare>. Some states are slow in reporting inspection results. The national website updates monthly, therefore there could be a time lag of a few weeks.

A copy of the last report will always be available in the facility, even though it may not yet be posted on the website.

CHAPTER 7

HOSPITAL DISCHARGE

Having an elderly loved one in the hospital is stressful. Compounding your worry about their recovery are the long hours at the bedside, cafeteria food and sitting, even sleeping, for hours on sparse hospital furniture. Now, emotionally drained, physically exhausted and mentally dull, the patient's family is often stretched further by a discharge notice which seems to conflict with the patient's welfare. Advocates can take comfort in the knowledge of their ultimate authority to authorize their loved one's discharge and that there are clear medical standards to determine whether their patient is ready for discharge. It is helpful to understand how hospitals' quick discharge mindset evolved.

Historically, Medicare paid hospitals a set amount based on the patient's diagnosis. Whether a patient received four days of care or ten days of care, the hospital's base payment was the same. So if a diagnosis allotted six days of care, and the patient was discharged within four days, the hospital kept the balance. Early discharges - before the patient received adequate treatment - became rampant. Over several years the Center for Medicare and Medicaid Services (CMS) tracked the consequences of early discharges. Their study found worsening health for patients, returns to the hospital and additional costs to Medicare.

The Affordable Care Act (ACA) attempted to correct the problems caused by early hospital discharges of Medicare patients by switching to a more traditional payment method, similar to daily rates. The transition and data collection of results are underway. We can expect hospital discharge planners and social workers to face a learning curve during this changeover. The effect on patients and families remains unclear.

Even if the ACA's changes achieve all the desired effects it still won't bring the interests of hospitals and patients into perfect alignment. The hospital's primary focus is on efficiency. This means making the bed available for the next person as soon as possible. To this end a referral pipeline has emerged. Staff often steers families toward an individual nursing home with whom they have a tacit arrangement - the facility receives lucrative Medicare referrals quickly and asks few questions. Often these arrangements result in hospitals discharging patients too soon and facilities agreeing to accept residents far too complex for their staffing and skill level. Sometimes nursing homes feel obligated to accept these patients because they fear the repercussions of losing future referrals from that hospital.

Whether going to a nursing home for the first time or returning after a hospital stay, patients often receive short notice of discharge and are pressured to choose a facility - sometimes within hours. Patients are often told, "Medicare won't pay anymore." This claim is almost always untrue and connected to hospital profits; the sooner the discharge, the more the hospital benefits. The first twenty-four to forty-eight hours involve significant diagnostic charges (labs, x-rays, scans). Thereafter, billable charges decrease. Hospital personnel are glad to coordinate a quick transfer through their pipeline with little effort (or deliberation) from the patient or responsible party. Transferring your loved one too early or to the wrong location can result in heartbreak from both treatment and financial standpoints.

You may never face more double talk than during transfers from the hospital to a nursing home (skilled nursing facility). Hospital and nursing home interests in this circumstance are *short-term* and financially motivated. Your interests are the *long-term* health and comfort of your loved one. Neither the hospital nor nursing home personnel know your loved one as you do: his or her personality, medical problems and finances. Before accepting their arrangements two considerations are of utmost importance; (1) is your patient ready to leave the hospital; and (2) which facility is best for your patient?

As payment transitions, it is helpful to know that the medical standard for hospital discharge has not changed, although it is often ignored. Even amidst urgent talk of discharge, a non-medical person is quite capable of applying the medical standards for discharge. Thus you can decide whether your loved one is ready for discharge. The medical standards for discharge are:

1. Stable vital signs (blood pressure, temperature, pulse and breathing rates) and no temperature elevation for twenty-four hours

2. An adequate method of taking nutrition and fluids, whether by mouth, tube feeding or intravenously
3. A pain management regimen in place which does not over sedate
4. A discharge plan in place, which assures safe, responsible care and assures continuation of the hospital treatment plan.

The method of payment does not figure into the above standards for discharge whether, private insurance, private pay, Medicare, Medicaid or a non-funded patient.

When deciding upon the best facility for your loved one, you may need twenty-four to forty-eight hours to make an informed decision. Questions loom large. Which facility uses Medicare payment for the best care and therapy immediately after hospitalization? Which facility best prepares residents to return to their own home or into permanent nursing home care where other payment sources become vital, i.e., Medicaid, private pay and long term care insurance?

The BE AWARE and BEWARE sections assure you of your rights and control. EXAMPLES follow.

BE AWARE
- Advocacy begins when your loved one is placed in a hospital bed, by finding out whether it is a hospital admission bed or an observation bed. The difference determines Medicare rehabilitation and skilled nursing home benefits.
    1. If a patient is *not* admitted in a hospital for three midnights they will not qualify for Medicare rehabilitation and skilled care in a nursing home. This care is contingent upon the Medicare Part A hospital inpatient admission.
    2. Sometimes patients are placed in hospital observation beds under Medicare Part B (outpatient care). Even though receiving the same treatment they are considered an outpatient leaving them ineligible for Medicare nursing home rehabilitation benefits, i.e., a skilled nursing facility (SNF) admission. Regardless of the type of health insurance, hospitals can bill observation patients for a larger share of the cost for any treatment and tests than if admitted as an inpatient.

3. Because observation patients receive the same care as admitted patients the best way to know whether a patient is an inpatient under Medicare Part A or an outpatient under Medicare Part B, is to ask. This is not a Medicare mistake, but a decision of the hospital and physician. Many patients lose valuable skilled nursing home benefits as a result. A 2017 regulation requires hospitals to notify patients when they are receiving observation care, but the notice can get lost.

- Before a hospitalized patient reaches the medical standard for discharge it is important to begin your own plan for leaving the hospital. Your best planning begins on admission day. Elderly patients usually benefit from a few days of therapy to regain strength and to recondition after a hospital stay. Receiving this rehabilitation is often dependent upon an advocate's voice.
- Many patients move from the hospital to a nursing home or skilled nursing facility with rehabilitation and a return to their home in mind. Others will remain as permanent residents. Payment source affects your facility choices. This chapter focuses on Medicare because it accounts for most nursing home patients' payment in the first twenty days after hospital discharge.
- Hospital personnel may guide you toward their own specially labeled in-hospital units, which focus on the lucrative first twenty days of Skilled Nursing Facility payment. Also, some rural hospitals tap into this first twenty days with a *swing bed* designation in order to tap into the Skilled Nursing Facility funding. Days spent in either setting is subtracted from the Medicare days available for payment in the nursing home or skilled nursing facility.
- It is helpful to remember the real value of Medicare - it pays for reasonable and necessary treatment when illness strikes. Whether a patient receives this care depends upon conscientious medical personnel and patient advocacy.
- Getting bogged down in the nuances of what Medicare pays for during hospitalization is a distraction from the real issue - is the patient reaching the discharge standards? When a patient meets the medical standard for discharge: stable vital signs, nutrition source, pain control and has a treatment plan (IV therapy, tube

feedings, physical therapy, etc.) in place, objection to the patient's discharge becomes unreasonable. It is reasonable to expect transfer to the facility of your choosing which may require time.
- Sometimes fast-tracked discharges leave a patient without any notice. There is a "fast appeal" process if the patient is unprepared to leave. Every Medicare patient should receive a copy of "<u>Important Message from Medicare</u>," which outlines the procedure for appealing when the patient is unprepared to leave. Within the information is a number for your Medicare Quality Improvement Organization (QIO), which will walk you through the process, but the call must be made immediately. The QIO can delay the discharge. The appeal cannot be used with observation stays (those billed under Medicare Part B).
- Those enrolled in Advantage (Medicare C) plans are dependent upon their group's negotiated contracts and case managers. Your hospital admission and discharge is largely in their hands. Still, Advantage plan patients familiar with discharge standards have enough knowledge to negotiate in an early discharge situation. The discharge standards are medical values unrelated to contracts and agreements between insurance plans and hospitals. The QIO appeal process is available to Medicare Advantage patients.
- The Affordable Care Act encouraged bundling- combining all services for an illness into one payment, i.e., hospital, doctors, skilled nursing care, rehabilitation centers, therapists, etc. So far, the concentration is on a few surgical procedures. The ACA's goal is improved quality and decreased costs over time. However, in 2018 the new CMS rules are decreasing the number of bundled contracts.
- A nursing home may send a resident to the hospital and then deny readmission when they are ready to return. Regardless of the reason, the facility will simply say, "We cannot meet the patient's needs." Sometimes there may not be an empty bed. A *bed hold* (prepayment to reserve the room) will avoid the "no bed available" problem but the return may still be rejected.

BEWARE

A hospitalized patient cannot be discharged or relocated without the responsible party's permission. Failure to *object* to a hospital discharge or transfer is considered agreement.

Beware of hospital personnel presenting themselves as a mouthpiece for Medicare, especially when their statements seem unreasonable. If you call Medicare to check on what they will or will not pay for, the answer is always, "What is reasonable and necessary." If a hospital calls Medicare about payment they are told the same thing. A few misrepresentations are noted below.

"Your Medicare won't pay any more. We'll be discharging you this afternoon."
- False! Medicare does not interfere in any way with the length of hospital admissions.
- The *Medical* Standard of Care for Hospital Discharge determines when you are ready for discharge.

"Your doctor said, 'you can go home.'"
- Was it really the doctor's idea? Hospital administrations influence doctors to hasten patient discharges. Professional pressure and threats to hospital privileges may result when one physician's patients are hospitalized longer than other physician's patients with similar medical problems.
- With the trend toward hospitalists (physicians employed or contracted by the hospital) now caring for most hospitalized patients, the advocacy of the private physician has been lost. The hospitalist's job and livelihood depend upon compliance with the employer's mindset.
- There is a hospital benefit to discharging a patient quickly before signs of complications develop. If a problem arises different from the admission diagnosis the payment for treating the new problem will be less than if the patient is discharged and then returns with the problem as a new diagnosis. Example: The patient who is hospitalized for pneumonia and suffers a heart attack the day before discharge. If the patient had been discharged and returned to the hospital with a heart attack, Medicare's reimbursement would be greater.

- The longer a patient stays in the hospital, the greater the risk of complications, especially avoidable problems such as infections, falls and medication errors which delay the discharge.
- After writing their order to discharge a patient, doctors generally defer to hospital staff for transfer options.

"We called your nursing home and your bed is waiting. We'll be calling the ambulance to take you back."

- Not so fast. The discharge is your call, not the hospitals. Remember the nursing home/skilled nursing facility is not equipped or staffed to care for patients requiring many hours of care or supervision. Consider the following questions before you consent:
    1. Does the patient have an adequate nutrition and fluid source? Can they feed themselves? Do they have new tube feedings?
    2. Does the patient have a pain management plan which the nursing home can continue? Has this routine been effective for at least twenty-four hours?
    3. If a patient needs physical, occupational or speech therapy has the treatment begun prior to discharge?
    4. Consider very carefully changes in activity and functional level. Has a patient who previously walked been out of bed? Does the patient need help getting to the bathroom? Have they become incontinent? Do they have sores on their skin? Have they developed other medical problems during hospitalization such as an infection or an allergic reaction?
    5. As a patient or caretaker use your judgment. Can the nursing home/skilled nursing facility provide the increased attention and care the resident will need after this hospitalization?

"Medicare tells us they won't pay for the hospital anymore but you still need a lot of specialized care. We'd like to move you to our hospital unit where we have therapy and nurses specially trained to take care of your individual needs."

- Remember, Medicare does not interfere in any way with determining the length of your hospital stay. However, when

transferred to their hospital skilled nursing unit a few days early, the hospital benefits by maximizing the hospital payment and a new Medicare reimbursement stream is triggered for skilled nursing care. Creative names can be misleading: subacute, acute skilled, transitional, etc. The Medicare billing is submitted as a skilled nursing facility-the same as a nursing home, and is paid 100 percent for 20 days.
- Consider the impact of using these few (20 days of 100 percent) prime Medicare payment days on later nursing home placement. For a new nursing home patient finding a good place may be more difficult. For a returning nursing home patient there may be little eligibility left for therapy and rehabilitation.
- The hospital skilled unit follows the routines of hospital care whereas the nursing home skilled care is more focused on functional level and returning to social activities, dining room, crafts, church services and group activities.
- Both settings provide therapy by licensed therapists.
- Marketing persons, discharge planners and social workers use the term "rehab" loosely when referring patients to these skilled units whether in the hospital or nursing home. Actual rehabilitation facilities provide care under a different license and patients must be strong enough to participate in therapy for six to eight hours daily—usually an impossibility for nursing home candidates.
- Long Term Acute Care (LTAC) may be needed for a patient requiring complex and extended care such as IV therapy, ventilator, wound care and difficult treatments. This is a separate Medicare admission and billing situation.

EXAMPLE: This instance of conflicting interest between a hospital and nursing home illustrates unnecessary stress and uncertainty heaped upon a family.

While employed by a large San Antonio nursing home, I received a Saturday morning message from a hospital; they were returning one of our residents, Mr. Guerra. He entered the hospital two weeks previously after suffering a heart attack. While there he caught a severe intestinal infection. Our facility kept up to date on his progress and anticipated he might be returning during the next week. If his intestinal symptoms were not resolved, his return could be problematic and costly: isolation supplies, private room, special diet and extra staffing hours. A family conference was scheduled for Monday to determine their expectations and if the facility could meet those needs.

Around noon, I notified the hospital case manager, "We cannot accept Mr. Guerra back into the facility until after a family conference on Monday."

She asked, "Why haven't you already had the conference?"

"We didn't expect him to return until next week. I'm sorry for..."

She interrupted, "I will be reporting this to my supervisor and the hospital administrator. Every other nursing home takes their patients back."

"I didn't say 'we won't take him back.' We just need to . . ."

A louder interruption, "You tell Medicare and Medicaid you can take care of patients and then you tell me you can't take care of Medicare patients?"

"I don't think there will be a problem. We may need to move patients so we can set up an isolation room. What about his infection?"

Her rising decibels and message surprised me. "I'm reminding you, we send a lot of patients to your facility. If you can't take care of patients we'll send them elsewhere!"

Within an hour Mr. Guerra's son, Rudy, called. "I'm worried. They say they're sending him back to the nursing home. I don't understand. On Thursday, the doctor told me 'he has an intestinal infection and he's not doing well.' On Friday his nurse said, 'he'll be in the hospital at least three more days to treat his infection.' Then the doctor called this morning and said, 'he'll be going back to the nursing home right away, we're removing his IV and catheter.'"

I said, "Rudy, they won't be sending your dad back today. I've talked with the hospital."

"Dad's so weak. He can't eat or drink anything. I'd like for him to get better before he comes back to the nursing home."

"We want your dad back in the nursing home, but not until he can eat and drink and his infection is under control."

"I understand, but what can I do? Dad can't even get out of bed now."

"Rudy, just remind the hospital and your insurance (a Medicare Advantage Plan) of their responsibility to make sure your dad is stable before he's discharged. He must be able to eat and drink before he leaves. Do not assume any responsibility for taking your dad out of the hospital before you're satisfied he is stable. Do not sign any papers."

"Okay."

"Remember your care plan meeting on Monday so we can plan for your dad."

Mr. Guerra returned to the nursing home on Tuesday.

EXAMPLE: A typical hospital attempt to shuffle an unstable patient from one Medicare program to another for the hospital's financial benefit.

The premature transfer of an unstable, hospitalized patient back to a nursing home is all too familiar. As a Director of Nursing for skilled nursing facilities, I often struggled to care for patients discharged from the hospital far too soon. Scant nursing home resources and short staffing ratios were never meant to attend to acutely ill, unstable patients. While working in positions responsible for discharge planning and quality assurance audits, I learned hospitals have obligations to fulfill prior to any discharge: 1) stable vital signs, 2) nutrition and fluid source, 3) pain control 4) safe, responsible care after discharge. Still, I was not prepared for a hospital's premature and dogged attempts to discharge my mother.

On December 23 Mother fell while serving fellow nursing home residents' coffee at their evening meal. She suffered a broken hip and uncontrolled pain in the emergency room. Dementia prevented her from understanding instructions and complicated her care. I explained the large amount of anti-anxiety medication she received routinely at the nursing home and asked for the medication to be continued. The emergency room physician declined to order the medication, but agreed to order a consultation with her gerontologist (Dr. G.).

The pain medication he ordered was not effective. A call to the doctor and increased dosage helped very little. She was transferred to her room whimpering and crying. After a sleepless night she was taken to surgery early the next morning, December 24. The nurse caring for her in the post anesthesia unit (recovery room) told me, "Her pain is severe and very difficult to manage. She doesn't comprehend anything. I called the doctor for stronger pain medicine."

During the day and throughout the night she refused food and spit out liquids. Her fitful sleep was limited to twenty or thirty minutes after receiving intravenous pain medication. Even then, she mumbled incoherently and picked at the air.

The orthopedic (bone) surgeon visited before breakfast on December 25. I asked him to order her anti-anxiety medication. He agreed, but did not do so. Instead he charted, "Confused at night. Usual for her." Family members provided constant bedside attention for her own safety: climbing out of bed, scratching at her dressing and pulling out tubes. Our presence assured she received pain medication on schedule; Mother was unable to ask. We struggled through another night of her confusion.

On the morning of December 26 the surgeon again arrived before breakfast. I told him of Mother's anxiety and pain and again requested her nursing home medication. He simply documented in his progress notes, "Confused this am. ? normal for patient."

By mid-morning Ann, a social worker, greeted me. "I wanted to let you know I'm making arrangements to transfer your mother back to the nursing home. I checked with her skilled nursing facility and she has a bed on reserve . . ." While Ann authoritatively ticked through her discharge checklist my mind wandered to Mother's pitiful moaning. She lay on the bed between us, oblivious to our conversation and relentlessly grabbing imagined objects from the air. "The ambulance will be arriving at 2:30 this afternoon. Do you have any questions?"

"I can't consent to Mother's transfer until she's seen by her gerontologist. I think she has an order for that consultation. Mother's not eating. She won't drink anything. Her pain is not under control. I will only agree to her discharge when the gerontologist feels the nursing home can manage all these problems."

"I'll check on the gerontology consult," Ann said.

On the morning of December 27 the surgeon visited and stood at the foot of mother's bed long enough to tell my son, "Mrs.

Vance's surgical status is stable." Then he charted, "Very confused and demented. Ortho stable, will transfer."

Dr. G. arrived soon thereafter and called with her findings. "Your mother is experiencing acute delirium. I've ordered lab and X-rays as well as a change in pain medication. I added Ativan to her medicines but it will be a while before we see improvement." Ativan was the nursing home medication I began asking for in the emergency room.

Ann returned mid-afternoon. "We would like to transfer your Mother to the ARU, our acute rehabilitation unit, where they have specialized nurses and a rehabilitation program."

Her message was code for moving mother from hospital charges to a unit which would begin billing Medicare for skilled nursing facility care. They would use the best twenty days of her Medicare Skilled Nursing Facility benefits and leave her with diminished rehabilitation possibilities when she returned to her nursing home. Most importantly, Mother needed hospital care, not rehab or nursing home care. Her welfare did not figure into any of Ann's proposals.

I answered, "Well, Mother's still really sick. She's not stable. Her pain is not controlled. How can she participate in a rehab program? She screamed bloody murder when the physical therapist tried to exercise her good leg (the no surgery leg). She's still not eating. She spits out any liquid we put in her mouth. No, I don't want her moved."

Ann returned later, "I'm sorry we won't be able to transfer your mother. There are no vacancies in the ARU."

Mother suffered a massive heart attack in the early morning hours of December 28. During the day she seemed weaker and in a deep sleep, arousing only to signal pain by grabbing her hip, moaning and grimacing.

On December 29 the gerontologist said, "Your mother's heart condition is worse. She is at risk for another heart attack, but she couldn't survive if that happens. I think we should make her a *No Code* status. I will continue treating her medical problems."

"I agree, totally," I said. The doctor ordered *Do Not Resuscitate*.

On the morning of December 30, the phone rang as I slipped into bed, tired after sitting with mother during the night.

The voice began, "I'm Doctor M., I'm seeing Dr. G's patients today. Your sister tells me I should talk with you about your mother's care."

"Yes, that's correct."

"Your mother needs to be put on hospice care."

"Why hospice?" I asked.

"Because she has a urinary tract infection. If we treat the infection she might live a few more days, but it really won't make any difference. She is still terminal so I'm going to put her on hospice."

"Do not order hospice," I replied.

"I've already written the order."

"Then you need to write an order to 'Discontinue Hospice,'" I replied.

"Why don't you want hospice?"

"Because, I want Dr. G's treatment continued."

"We can continue the treatment and just put her on hospice for pain management."

"Pain management? What kind of pain management?" I asked.

"We can give her stronger pain medicine if she's on hospice."

"What kind of medicine?"

"It's complicated, but just stronger pain medicine," he answered.

"Who will be giving this medicine?"

"The nurses."

"The same nurses she has now?" I asked.

"Yes."

"I fail to see how changing Mother to hospice will help her. When the nurses give the medicine Dr. G ordered on time it works well. She has horrible pain when it's delayed. So, I don't see why she needs a stronger medication when there is no guarantee the same nurses will give the hospice medicine when she needs it."

"Well, the hospice medicine lasts longer so you don't have to call the nurses so often."

I was slow to answer, "No hospice. Absolutely no hospice."

"What do you have against hospice?"

I struggled to control my anger and tears. "Doctor, I'd like to have a philosophical discussion with you about hospice when I'm not so tired. But for now, no hospice for Mother."

"Do you want her urinary infection treated?"

I hesitated. What to do? *Treatment means IV antibiotics, more sticks in her delicate veins, more medication side effects, more discomfort.* "Don't treat the infection," I answered.

Around six p.m. that evening I was opening my car door to leave the hospital. Someone yelled my name from across the parking lot. *Did something happen to Mother while I was in the elevator?*

A young lady rushed toward me and introduced herself as the hospice nurse. "Your sister told me you were just leaving the hospital. I wanted to talk to you about hospice for your mother."

"I've already told Dr. M. we don't want hospice."

"Well, he wrote an order for hospice. We can offer many services for your mother and the family."

"I'm really tired. I'm on my way home."

"That's one way hospice can help you. We can send sitters for your mother and give the family some rest."

"Our family feels better sitting with Mother ourselves," I said.

"I have the paperwork here. You can sign it now and we can get hospice started right away."

"No. I will not sign anything now. You can check with me tomorrow."

"Okay," she said. "We'll contact you tomorrow."

I returned to Mother's room to update my sister. Mother dozed peacefully and Sister was occupied with a book. *Not much need for hospice here.*

The hospice social worker called at 7:30 a.m. the next morning, December 31. I listened patiently as she sympathized with Mother's condition and ticked through hospice benefits—medical, financial, and family support.

I said, "I don't believe Mother needs anything you've described: sitters, a chaplain, more medication, a hospice nurse, a hospice physician? We're satisfied with Dr. G's care."

"Dr. G's out of town for the holidays," she answered.

"Mother had major surgery seven days ago, a massive heart attack three days ago. We understand she may die, but she deserves a chance to get better. Hospice does not offer that chance. Again, my answer is: No hospice. We will wait for Dr. G. to return."

Mother succumbed to heart failure on January 1.

Mother's hospital experience happens all too often. This cold and indifferent shift of responsibility is quite profitable for the hospital. But it's risky for the patient and presents serious, sometimes dangerous, challenges for care at the nursing home/skilled nursing facility.

Like most families we didn't question additional Medicare charges, but we did doubt the benefit to Mother. Think, for just a moment about the hospitals' proposed changes. The first December 27 proposed discharge back to the nursing home meant savings for the hospital. The second December 27 proposed discharge to the hospital's ARU meant the same savings plus increased funds from a new Medicare revenue stream. The December 30 proposed discharge to the hospital's hospice meant sizeable (very sizeable) new Medicare revenue within a few hours for consultations, assessments, medications, etc. In fact, all the proposed changes would have resulted in less care. Mother was acutely ill. What she needed was more care.

References

HOSPITAL DISCHARGES: Kaiser Health News reference: "It's a mistake to rely on hospital staff to ensure that things go smoothly; medical centers' interests (efficiency, opening up needed beds, maximizing payments, avoiding penalties) are not necessarily your interests (recovering as well as possible, remaining independent and easing the burden on caregivers)." Kaiser Health News

AFFORDABLE CARE ACT CHANGES: The ACA initiated complex changes in the Medicare and Medicaid payment systems. The turn was toward quality with data collection used to categorize performance. After identifying the adverse consequences of early discharges, CMS began tracking hospitals with high percentages of readmissions within thirty days of discharge. Also, CMS followed nursing homes with large numbers of residents sent back to the hospital within thirty days after they arrived from the hospital.

The ACA pursued changes by modestly reducing Medicare payments to hospitals with high percentages of readmissions and extra financial support for hospitals that develop ways to improve quality of care.

In a September 15, 2016 report CMS noted declining hospital readmissions. Whether quality of care has improved is still undetermined.

DENIED NURSING HOME READMISSION: A nursing home may decide not to accept a former resident when they are discharged from the hospital. Some of the unstated reasons are behavior problems, high cost patients (supplies, supplements and staffing) and problem families. The stated reason for not accepting the patient will usually be, "Our facility is unable to provide for the patient's needs."

A nursing home may send a resident to the hospital with the intent of denying readmission. It is easier to deny entry back into the facility than use involuntary discharges or evictions from within.

The nursing home can be forced to justify their denied readmission by filing a complaint with the state's regulatory agency. The complaint will be judged on whether other residents in the facility require similar care. The decision will come long after the resident's placement in another facility.

BED HOLD: A daily rate charged during the time a resident is not in the facility. Many facilities charge the full room price, others only a portion of the rate. Without a bed hold you will probably be asked to remove your loved one's personal items to allow the facility to admit another resident. In some instances they may store the resident's possessions. If another bed is available when the resident returns they will face adjustment to another room, perhaps a different unit with different nurses and a new roommate. Only a few states provide Medicaid funding for bed holds or room holds. Medicare pays nothing on bed holds. Payment is predominantly from private money.

The Nursing Reform Act of 1987 guaranteed that a Medicaid resident's bed be held in the nursing home for one week during hospitalization. The regulation is mostly ignored.

SWING BED: The term Medicare uses to describe a hospital room that can switch from acute care (hospital) status to skilled care (nursing home). These hospitals are located in rural areas and are considered critical access hospitals (CAH), that is, they provide care not easily available in the area. Most rural communities large enough to have a hospital also have at least one nursing home providing Medicare skilled care. Medicare days spent in a hospital swing bed are no longer available in the nursing home. The hospitals typically use most of the twenty days that Medicare pays at 100 percent and then seek nursing home placement.

https://www.cms.gov/Outreach-and-Education/Medicare-Learning-Network-MLN/MLNProducts/downloads/SwingBedFactsh

Nursing Homes Turn to Eviction to Drop Difficult Patients: *The Associated Press*, May 8, 2016.

CHAPTER 8
ADMISSION DAY

Moving into a nursing home is a sea change in our life cycle: a shift from independence to reliance, strange surroundings, a horde of new faces, institutional routines, a stranger for a roommate and other aggravations.

Remembering the necessity of nursing home care tends to resolve gloom linked to the move. Looking forward, you and your loved one have every reason to expect safe, kind, around-the-clock care. Most residents are apprehensive on admission day, but experienced nurses and nurses' aides can help ease the stress.

A session in the business office will precede any introduction to the nursing staff or a roommate. Twenty-plus pages requiring initials and signatures are usually presented as a necessity ("just routine" is the usual explanation) at a time when new residents and their families are winding down a stressful journey.

The papers are a legal contract crafted to (1) secure payment and (2) construct a wall protecting the facility from responsibility and lawsuits. There is enough buried in the contract for attorneys to recommend obtaining a copy for legal review before signing. Their good advice does not take into consideration the time needed to review and analyze—an impossible luxury for the resident facing a stack of papers on admission day. Most families are emotionally and physically drained. They have neither the time nor money for consulting attorneys.

Who signs the papers? The resident's own signature will avoid future entanglements. An alternate is needed only if the new resident is physically unable to sign or has been declared incompetent by a physician or court. "Representative" appears on most documents, but the terms and legal effects vary by state. Generally, Representative indicates the contact person, not necessarily a Power of Attorney or Medical Power of Attorney, but a substitute decision maker.

I wish there were reasonable bypasses for the legal and financial traps contained in admission contracts. But the realities are: a loved one needs care, any facility can reject their admission if you do not sign the contract as presented, you cannot expect to find a better admission contract at another facility. Working through this first nursing home experience may leave you exhausted, but I offer the best of survival tactics - choose your battles.

The BE AWARE and BEWARE sections offer further explanation and insight into admission day. EXAMPLES follow.

BE AWARE
- The admission contract and paperwork are the same for short stay rehabilitation and permanent residents.
- Admission papers are contracts and will be used as legal instruments when problems arise. Much is written about securing copies for attorney review prior to admission, which reminds me that nursing homes and lawyers mix like oil and water. Obtaining a copy of the nursing home contract before admission might be possible, but would also be an exception. Such a request could trigger alarms causing the facility to reconsider accepting the resident, i.e., attorneys and troublemakers.
- The usual course is cautious signing on admission day. Contracts are rather standard, varying only slightly from one facility to another. The facility spokesperson will ask you to bring several legal and medical documents. I hope you will read the following chapter before producing anything other than identification, insurance cards and a designation of representative decision maker. Often Living Wills, Do Not Resuscitate orders, Directives to Physicians and Advance Directives become problematic in nursing homes. I suggest you leave them at home, available for future use.
- Almost all facilities have added arbitration clauses to admission contracts. This agreement forces any dispute, even wrongful death, into arbitration, whereby a supposedly neutral arbitrator is chosen by the nursing home and acts as judge and jury to determine nursing home responsibility. The resident is denied their day in court, and the records are sealed from public scrutiny. Options for rejecting arbitration clauses are limited. The nursing home can still refuse your admission and finding a facility without the clause is probably impossible.

- There are suggestions of marking through and initialing portions of the contract you do not agree with. The reality remains that nursing homes choose whom to admit and your loved one has not yet been admitted.
- There is a lot buried in the contract's complex list of decisions. A few of the determinations you will need to make are:
  1. Release of Information approval—needed to secure medical information and bill insurance, Medicare and Medicaid.
  2. Name your physician—you can continue with your own physician if he/she agrees. Expect the facility to suggest the services of their medical director.
  3. Designate a pharmacy—you have the option of using your own local pharmacy. Any hint of better service from their contracted pharmacy is a sales pitch.
  4. Photographic permission—a photo will be used to confirm resident identity for new and temporary employees giving medications and treatments, during disaster evacuations and runaway situations.
  5. Select a mortuary—prearrangements or a signed burial agreement are not necessary.
  6. Decide if the resident's clothing will be laundered by the facility or collected for the family to launder; laundry service is included in the daily rates.
  7. Agreement with smoking policies—some facilities refuse to accept new residents who smoke.
- A few facilities post admission contracts on their website. Given enough time you can also find sample contracts and attorney reviews by Googling: Nursing Home Admission Contracts National. The pitfall is discovering ominous details and realizing your ability to challenge them is limited. After all, your first concern is finding care for your loved one.
- You should receive a copy of the Resident's Bill of Rights.
- A resident or responsible party cannot be expected to understand and remember the huge volume of information in the admission paperwork. Be sure to get a copy of the signed contract and review it after a few weeks rest.
- Staff will try to match roommates of equal functional level and compatibility. An example is avoiding placement of an alert,

talking resident with someone who is comatose. When the facility is full, initial choices may be limited, but it remains the nursing home's duty to find harmonious roommates.
- When you finally arrive at the new room, begin sizing up nursing staff. Look for the caring, respectful nurse or nurse's aide . . . those taking enough time to communicate with your loved one. You will be compiling a mental list of employees who will be helpful in the future.
- Closet space is limited. A few seasonal clothes are a good start. Staff can help you decide on further choices.
- All personal items, including clothing, will need to be labeled with the resident's name.
- An inventory of possessions brought to the nursing home is tedious but necessary to identify lost items and verify that the resident arrived with the articles.
- The new resident will need an adjustment period of several days. Visits at all hours by the responsible party will reassure and comfort an alert, responsible resident. Unannounced appearances around the clock are even more important for those who are mentally or physically unable to recognize and communicate problems.
- Roommates often become complimentary companions. However, if they are incompatible, the old roommate has a right to stay and the new resident moves.

BEWARE
- Amid vague variations of Responsible Party, Representative, Surrogate, Decision Maker, Guardianship, etc., nursing homes have sometimes buried agreements of personal guarantee for payment even though it is against federal law. To clarify your status, write "signing as agent of resident" after your signature.
- It has long been illegal for a nursing home to require a resident to assign any income or property to the nursing home. The nursing home cannot become representative payee for Social Security checks. Residents usually maintain a personal bank account from which the nursing home is paid monthly.
- A nursing home cannot require a family member to guarantee payment of the resident's bill. Federal Law, Title 42, US Code Sec. 483. 12(d)(2), says, "The facility must not require a third

party guarantee of payment to the facility as a condition of admission."
- Any extra documents not a part of the original contract may be agreements to invalidate parts of the twenty-page contract. An example is changing financial responsibility to the responsible party, family or friend signing the contract.
- Medicaid eligibility does not interfere with a resident's right to maintain his/her own bank account. Medicaid residents' portion of payment (applied income) will be paid from the personal account. Pension checks and Social Security deposits continue into the resident's bank account.
- Some facilities limit the number of Medicaid residents. They can ask if a resident is eligible for Medicare or Medicaid. They cannot request personal financial information in order to assure that the resident is not eligible for Medicaid or will not apply for Medicaid benefits in the near future.
- Facilities can require a deposit for privately paying residents, but cannot ask for deposits on Medicare and Medicaid residents.
- The facility may charge privately paying residents (non Medicare or Medicaid) any amount for room and services, but must notify in advance, according to the admission contract.
- Hints of preferred treatment in return for donations for facility projects are illegal enough to land the administrator in jail.
- Do not leave anything of value with the resident. The admission contract included a clause releasing the facility of responsibility for loss or theft.

EXAMPLE: How competent staff resolved a roommate conflict on Mother's first nursing home admission. The facility's responsibility is to remove a resident from an unsafe situation.

Mother half-heartedly followed the nurse into her room where an angry roommate greeted her. She waved, her arms toward the door and shouted, "No, no, no. Go, go!" After the nurse's persuasion the roommate moved to a corner chair. She sat quietly, but defiantly, arms crossed, while I hung mother's clothes and arranged a few personal articles in the bedside stand.

The nurse said, "It's almost dinner time. I'll introduce Mrs. Vance to the other residents." I left Mother sitting woefully in the other corner chair, but felt she was in good hands.

I returned the next morning to find her moved to a distant room on another hall. A nurse explained, "We thought the other roommates language was abusive so we moved Mrs. Vance out of the situation. Don't worry, it was all in Spanish and your mother didn't understand a word."

Thus began a deep friendship with a new roommate, Stella. Mutual appreciation of their circumstances grew by leaps and bounds. Each perceived themselves to be the other's keeper throughout Mother's stay.

EXAMPLE: An upsetting admission day and illustration of the facility's responsibility to find compatible room placements.

Mother arrived at her second nursing home amid the upheaval of personnel changes. The chaos aggravated her confusion and signaled problems to come.

The admission clerk led us to Mother's room. "Someone will be with you shortly."

Mother sat in the cramped corner of her new room. With no other chair in sight, I perched on the bed. We were tired and glad to rest after the long paper signing process.

A man and woman dressed for business entered the room, interrupting our quiet. The unbending, oversized lady extended her hand to mother. *This must be a nurse. She's using the universal medical gesture to evaluate Mother's awareness.* Mother appropriately extended her hand.

She said, "I'm Doris Johnson the Director of Nursing, but you won't be seeing me again. I just received a promotion and will be working as a consultant for all our corporation's facilities in Texas."

The nattily attired young man kept his distance. "Mrs. Vance, welcome to our home. I'm John Anderson, just the temporary administrator, so I'll be replaced in about a week." *No extended hand here.*

Mother strained to comprehend. I nodded. Their departure was as stiff as their arrival. *Well, that's the way it goes in this business, incompetents move up the corporate ladder quickly. High heels, dangling jewelry and designer nails tell me she has no intention of tending to residents.*

Mother stiffened her back. Wide-eyed, she moved to the front six inches of her chair and blurted, "What the hell was that woman talking about?"

"Mother, I don't know but we've got trouble of our own. We can't be worried about that woman."

"Well, ain't that the damn truth! Honey, call Dick, I need to get the hell outta here." For many years mother had depended on Dick, her son-in-law, to resolve serious problems. I will not be calling him today.

Nurses and nursing assistants arrived within a few minutes. The adjoining bed was empty. Staff said the resident was in the hospital. Mother asked the nurses to call Dick, but they deferred that decision to me. I diverted her attention to helping me unpack and arrange her new room. She seemed satisfied and looked forward to a grandson delivering her TV.

I left, but called near bedtime. The nurse reported, "She enjoyed supper. She's just visiting with everybody."

A nurse summoned as I entered the next morning. "We may have to transfer Mrs. Vance to a locked facility where they can manage her aggressive behavior."

"What?"

"Well, the lady across the hall was crying during the night. Mrs. Vance kept yelling, 'Shut up.' When she didn't quit, your mother went to her bedside and yelled."

"Did Mother hit the other resident or hurt her."

"No, she just yelled."

"Surely, you can find another room on another hall where Mother can't hear the crying." *What about the crying resident? Did she get any help? She must have been suffering from anxiety or pain?*

Mother was moved to a distant room on another hallway. She and her new roommate developed another lasting friendship. I learned to depend on Vala's observations and insight into the staff's care and interaction with Mother.

References

In the late 1990s plaintiff attorneys realized that nursing home residents have value. Lawsuits identifying preventable harm to residents forced facilities to improve care through court judgments and public awareness of trials. Care improved as a result. Within a few years the industry began quietly adding forced arbitration clauses to admission contracts. In arbitration cases the mediator, chosen by the facility, rarely rules in favor of the resident. Additionally, the cost to the resident including the mediator's fee is usually well into five figures. The mediation proceedings and records are sealed from public scrutiny. The nursing home industry breathed a sigh of relief and returned to previous violations of nursing home standards of care. Resident care deteriorated.

When the Center for Medicare and Medicaid Services (CMS) issued new rules barring forced arbitration from nursing home contracts beginning November 28, 2016, the industry trade group, The American Health Care Association (AHCA) succeeded in securing an injunction blocking implementation of the rule from a Mississippi judge. Now the Trump administration is pushing to scrap the rule change, which will result in a return to forced arbitration in nursing home conctracts.

CHAPTER 9
ADVANCE DIRECTIVES

Most of us feel a heavy responsibility to define and document our wishes for medical care. Instructions for end-of-life medical care receive heightened attention during transition to a nursing home. It is important to consider how a facility's interest in these instructions often conflicts with a resident's well-being.

One of the first questions asked when signing the admission paperwork is, "Do you want resuscitative measures if we find you not breathing or without a heartbeat?" The reference is to Do Not Resuscitate (DNR) or Cardiopulmonary Resuscitation (CPR). The question evokes images of nurses pumping on a patient's chest, attempts to restore breathing and ultimately life support systems. Many will readily verbalize some variation of, "No, let me go in peace."

The next question will be "Do you have a signed directive?" This reference is to prepared documents that become effective if you are mentally or physically unable to make decisions. The document titles vary by state: Advanced Health Care Directive, Living Will, Personal Directive, Advanced Decision, Medical Power of Attorney, Healthcare Proxy and many others. All are lumped into the term *advance directives*.

Sometimes advance directives are simple in that they provide only one instruction. More recently advance directives progressed to extensive check lists directing care for multiple options: medications, feeding tubes, blood transfusions, breathing machines and much more. We are conditioned to find comfort in preparing these documents. They guide doctors and relieve our family of burdensome decisions. However, within nursing homes the intent of these directives is often altered to fit into physicians' personal philosophies.

An example is the Do Not Resuscitate (DNR) and No Cardiopulmonary Resuscitation (NO CPR) instructions. Both are used often and well understood by the public. They are also the directives most often hijacked by physicians in command of nursing home residents' medical care.

To individuals, the meaning of No CPR and DNR documents is pure and simple: *"If you find me not breathing and without a heartbeat, do not try to revive me."* That is what the document says. That is what it means. The medical meaning is the same and is usually referred to as the Code status.

If a resident has no directive saying "No CPR" or "DNR" all nursing homes and medical facilities will attempt to restore breathing and a heartbeat (resuscitation). Resuscitation is not a default position. Resuscitation is the *baseline standard for medical care*. If you do not want resuscitation you must put it in writing—DNR (Do Not Resuscitate) or No Cardiopulmonary Resuscitation (No CPR).

A No CPR or DNR does not mean you reject treatment for an illness such as infection, allergic reaction, stroke, heart attack, food poisoning or any other treatable condition. However, the most frequently asked question when nurses contact a physician about a new symptom or problem is, "What is the Code status?" Meaning: is there a DNR or No CPR document on this resident?

The No CPR or DNR instructions should not enter this conversation. Yet their presence often results in delayed treatment with a doctor ordering, "Call me back if he gets worse" or "Let's watch her for a while." A nurse would not be calling without a change in the resident's condition. In many instances the nurse is requesting an order to send the resident to the emergency room for a physician's examination.

The application of a doctor's personal philosophy to a No CPR or DNR often means delayed, inferior or no treatment. Token treatment such as a less effective antibiotic or just enough intervention to keep the doctor out of court is common. Some doctors are demeaning of nursing home residents' worth and treat them accordingly. A surprising number feel the residents have no value to society; too many resources are spent on nursing home care and; nursing home residents' quality of life is miserable and any medical care will only prolong their misery.

If the straightforward DNR or No CPR is hijacked so easily, imagine the possibilities for abuse in detailed directives. A resident's health and wellbeing can be adversely affected when doctors use advance directives to ignore symptoms or delay diagnosis and treatment.

Your loved one may spend years in a nursing home before facing end of life decisions. When there are no instructions (advance directives, No CPR/DNR) they are more likely to receive appropriate treatment during their journey. Weigh this against the rare instance of finding a resident not breathing or without a heartbeat.

Concern about end of life medical care and futile attempts to keep someone alive are justified. However, in a nursing home the more urgent issue is securing minimal care for common, treatable illnesses.

There is a solution. Consider leaving all advanced directives at home. You can protect your wish not to be on life support or any other treatment by discussing your wishes with a family member or friend and preparing a legal document naming that person as your agent. The agent becomes your spokesperson if you are unable to make decisions. They can present your advance directives when needed, perhaps within a few days of imminent death.

The BE AWARE and BEWARE sections offer additional insight and suggestions for improving your chances of having wishes fulfilled. EXAMPLES of this unfortunate mindset follow. Many others happen every day.

BE AWARE
- It is helpful to remember that treatment can be stopped at any time but the disaster of *not* receiving resuscitation may be irreversible. Your agent or spokesperson has the ability to apply your wishes to any treatment you would not wish.
- Attorneys recommend that beyond appointing an agent you can also name alternate agents in the event your agent is unable to make decisions.
- A resident may appear to be not breathing or not have a pulse in situations such as fainting, seizures, strokes and blood pressure changes. Most of these collapses are observed and treatment can be initiated without delay. The presence of a No CPR/DNR may slow down emergency interventions increasing the risk of brain damage if the resident arouses on his own. Treatment would be provided immediately if the resident did not have No CPR/DNR instructions.
- Even though a resident is alert and able to make decisions, treatment options may never be discussed if a physician

chooses to apply their own interpretation to advance directives. Examples are: choices for cancer treatment, heart problems, lung trouble, strokes, infections, blood disorders, etc.
- Rapid medical progress and our inability to predict future healthcare conditions create situations advance directives cannot foresee or tackle. For example: a healthcare directive may reject tube feedings, but an unforeseen disease can be treated and cured with a feeding tube inserted for one month and then removed.
- When facing mortality, residents often make swift adaptations favoring treatment rejected in their advance directives. Residents with "No hospitalization" directives often say, "Yes, send me to the hospital" when informed they are suffering a heart attack and could die.

BEWARE
- The No CPR/DNR question not only comes early in the nursing home admission process, it persists throughout the resident's stay. Facilities are good at obtaining signed No CPR/DNR documents.
- Nursing homes prefer to have No CPR/DNRs and advance directives—they feel it makes them less liable for serious mistakes and resident injuries. Their defense attorneys have successfully distorted these instructions to mean the resident was responsible for an injury because the document limited the nursing home interventions.
- Even more disheartening is the takeover of the No CPR/DNRs intention by nursing home attorneys. Their argument in wrongful death cases: "The resident faced his mortality with the Do Not Resuscitate directive. You can't blame the nursing home. He knew he was going to die."
- Inferior medical practices are difficult for a person with no medical background to identify. It is especially tough for the elderly resident since most have high regard and trust of doctors. There is no peer review or oversight of nursing home doctors, therefore abuse of advance directives will continue.
- There is an effort toward Physician Orders for Life-Sustaining Treatment (POLST)—electronic physician orders which travel with a patient from beginning to end of an emergency situation.

The set of medical orders signed by the physician and patient or responsible party are accessed electronically and do not allow participation of an agent or designated decision maker. They are not legal documents, but simply physician's orders following the patient from one care setting to another. Medical personnel following POLST orders are protected from legal action if claiming they followed the orders in good faith.

EXAMPLE: A personal physician distorts the meaning of No CPR/DNR.

Agatha, an alert, frail eighty-year-old came to the nursing home because of extreme weakness. She kept falling at home and was at risk of serious injury. The new resident needed support when getting out of bed or walking. However, she was prideful and too independent to call the nurses for help.

During her first two weeks in the facility she fell numerous times. Nurses contacted the physician with each fall. On several occasions they requested an order to send her to the emergency room. They felt she needed to be checked for internal injury and broken bones.

The physician always refused the request, "She's a DNR. There's nothing to do."

She fell one weekend when her physician was off duty. The substitute physician ordered her transfer to the emergency room. Routine lab work revealed a critically low blood count with profound anemia. Agatha received blood transfusions in the emergency room and returned to the nursing home on an anemia treatment regimen.

There were no further falls. She returned to her own home and active social circle within two weeks.

EXAMPLE: A nursing home's overbearing pressure to obtain No CPR/DNR documents.

"Now, if we find Mrs. Vance not breathing, do you want heroic measures?" The question sprang up early during the signing of Mother's admission paperwork.

"If you find my mother not breathing, I want her resuscitated vigorously. I want EMS called immediately and I want her transported to the hospital," I replied.

The admissions clerk paused before coordinating a flip of her hair with a twist of her overstuffed, swivel chair to face Mother. I looked toward Mother. She sat hunched in a hard, straight-backed corner chair, bundled in her soft fleece jacket, arms folded across her chest and head bowed as she stared at the floor. The clerk proceeded as though I were not present or had not spoken.

"So, Mrs. Vance, do you want heroic measures?"

While I tried to gather a response, Mother replied in a weary monotone. "Dick takes care of my business. You have to ask him." She referred to my sister's husband.

"Mother is absolutely correct. You have Power of Attorney and Medical Power of Attorney designation in the paperwork, stacked on your desk. Nowhere has anyone indicated a Do Not Resuscitate status. Mother is to be resuscitated."

"Well, let's move along with this paperwork. Do you have a living will, Mrs. Vance?"

"Mother has no living will, no advanced directive and no prior instructions for your records. She does have a Power of Attorney and I am her designated spokesperson for the nursing home. We know her wishes. Our instructions to you are to treat any medical problems aggressively including resuscitation. Her Power of Attorney can be easily contacted for any other decisions. "Isn't that right Mother? They need to call Dick for trouble?"

"Yep. That's right. Call Dick."

The issue of DNR never went away during Mother's stay at this facility. It was the first concern addressed at care plan meetings. Her dementia was in the forefront when I received calls from psychiatric consultants and social workers. They suggested that I reconsider by gently posturing Mother's *quality of life* and avoiding the *heroics* of resuscitation as benevolent reasons to sign Do Not Resuscitate instructions.

In order to avoid confusion, I sent Mother's physician the following letter of explanation. She faxed it to the facility for inclusion in Mother's chart.

> Dr. _____, I just do not trust some alternate health care providers to treat Mother appropriately

in the presence of a "DNR". I've recently seen token treatment and absence of treatment for elderly nursing home patients based on their "no code" status. Certainly, your good judgment will always prevail, but in your absence, who knows what philosophical nut may be taking care of her.

My experience with the realities of No CPR/DNR and advance directive abuse by health care providers led me to this firm refusal to provide any directive for specific care. When there are no instructions, there is no opportunity for philosophical interpretation. A physician is more likely to treat the resident according to established medical practice.

EXAMPLE: How a physician's personal views impacted his professional practice.

I was once naïve enough to think I could reason with a physician caring for a severely malnourished resident. He had refused other nurses' requests for nutritional supplements and high protein snacks.

The resident fell, broke her hip and lay on her kitchen floor for three days before being found. During that time Miss Emma was unable to move. The constant pressure of her body weight against the hard floor caused large sores on her hip, shoulder and foot. After surgical repair of her hip she came to the nursing home for treatment of sores penetrating into muscle.

Healing would require huge amounts of nutrients, especially protein and calories. Her own body's reserves were used up rapidly leaving her malnourished. It was impossible for her to consume enough nutrients in regular meals to support healing. Nurses requested doctor's orders for supplements, high protein shakes and special foods with concentrated calories. All required a physician's order. He refused.

After three weeks, Miss Emma remained alert and totally engaged in her care but every day she seemed weaker. Treatment of the worsening sores was painful. Bone was visible in the depths of her sores.

I reasoned that her physician surely did not understand the full picture of Miss Emma's deterioration. I interrupted his Sunday morning rounds and asked him to look at her sores. He didn't have time and seemed a bit agitated, nor did he respond to my description of her deteriorating wounds. As he thumbed through her chart I reminded him of her pain as well as delightful conversations the nurses enjoyed with her.

The usual and accepted treatment for Miss Emma's sores was lab work, high-protein, high-calorie supplements and possibly a feeding tube for a few months. I asked him to consider this treatment.

"Of course not, she's a DNR," he snapped. Miss Emma signed a DNR the day she arrived. I pictured her being whizzed through the admission process geared to quickly gain signatures. I doubted she received any meaningful explanation of what she was signing.

As I tried to discuss the absolute meaning of a DNR his real reasoning surfaced. The doctor felt too much money and resources were spent on end-of-life care. The money would be better spent on the beginning of life. He considered everyone in the nursing home an end of life patient. "I'm doing my part to at least limit end of life expense." I sat stunned as he progressed to near rage, slammed the chart across the desk and stormed away.

I thought of the possibilities if Miss Emma had received nutritional support when she arrived: her sores would have healed; with the help of therapy she could have walked again . . . maybe even returned home. All combined were far less costly than the extended expense of treating her sores. Instead, Miss Emma suffered malnutrition, dehydration, huge infected sores and unnecessary pain.

Then I considered how denying Miss Emma her opportunity for improved health affected the doctor: he still charged Medicare, Medicaid and privately for visits to Miss Emma and other residents— he was the attending physician for eighty percent of the residents in our building, one of the largest facilities in the state; he still received a substantial monthly sum as the facility's medical director; he continued to work quick rounds into weekends allowing him to maintain private practice office hours during the week. As medical director, he provided the final review of all medical practice within the building. There would be no chance of peer review or oversight of his negligent application of the DNR.

Within a few days of our conversation he ordered hospice care—an added shield against any further questions.

EXAMPLE: How prior written directives can conflict with more immediate attitude changes about death.

Most nursing home residents speak of being "ready to go." They express wishes of limited treatment and often non-treatment. Verbalizations include prayers and requests to "just take me on home," meaning the hereafter. However, only a few residents continue the wish when facing reality.

My mother was typical. For years her conversations led to wishes of "going home to be with George." Tearful breakdowns tested the family's stamina with repetitions of "just let me go, I want to go, I'm ready."

During her nursing home stay I often brought her to my home for coffee and short visits. On one occasion she sat in her usual chair at the kitchen table. She had a view through the living room and into the bedroom. Mother's attention became fixed on my son sitting on the bedside.

He presented a miserable picture, having just returned from the hospital following sinus surgery. His coughing, spitting up blood, swollen face and painful groans elicited her concern. She sat upright, stiffened her back and strained for a better view.

Within a few minutes she pushed her untouched coffee aside. Eyes wide open she said, "Honey, you better take me back to my place. If I catch that stuff he's got, I won't last a week."

Recall of this event always provides our family a chuckle. Families and responsible parties would do well to remain flexible and mindful of residents' tendency to change their minds when confronting their own mortality.

References

"The most comprehensive health care planning you can do is to name an agent." Advocate Tony Chicotel staff attorney at California Advocates for Nursing Home Reform in San Francisco.

http://californiahealthline.org

CHAPTER 10

RESIDENT RIGHTS

An often overlooked aspect of nursing home life is the individual rights residents carry with them into the facility. "Resident's Rights" involves much more than the weighty decisions usually associated with the term: right to dignity, refuse feeding tubes, breathing tubes and resuscitation. Simple pleasures and small wishes also fall within the realm of resident's rights…perhaps a late bedtime, ice cream with every meal, a 3:00 a.m. phone call or a private place for conversation or sex. Plainly stated, residents do not give up their civilian rights when they enter a nursing home.

A copy of "Resident Rights" is provided to each new nursing home resident. Staff is trained during initial orientation and annually. Most facilities are flexible in honoring reasonable requests thus avoiding clashes stemming from resident's rights. Still, it often becomes the residents' or their advocates' task to assure that rights requests are acknowledged and fulfilled.

Nursing homes are responsible for each resident's health and safety. The facility has the right to decide whether a resident's request is unsafe or presents a health risk. If the nursing home determines a resident is claiming resident's rights in a dangerous way they will usually have the resident or responsible party sign a "Release of Responsibility" document for that particular activity. An example is a resident claiming the right to walk without a walker even though rickety on his feet. The document acknowledges the resident's claim of his right to walk without a walker, and states the facility is not responsible for injuries resulting from this decision, such as, falls, broken bones and death.

There are great variances in application of resident's rights across the industry. Flexible staffs focusing on resident's preferences and care usually find ways to accommodate individual requests without rights becoming an issue. Other facilities use resident's rights and release of responsibility documents excessively, and often as legal cover for their own failures.

Within a resident's right to a safe environment, lies the issue of verbal and physical abuse and neglect. Our humanity dictates nursing home residents' right to an abuse-free environment. Media reports of resident abuse stir our anger. All long-term care staff and administrators have strict rules for reporting incidents of abuse or suspected abuse to regulatory agencies and law enforcement. Episodes of abuse, including injuries, often go unreported thus leaving the nursing home's record clean and avoiding public scrutiny.

Further explanation and how to tackle resident rights and abuse incidents are provided in the BE AWARE and BEWARE sections. EXAMPLES follow. A copy of resident's rights is located in APPENDIX B.

BE AWARE
- The Nursing Home Reform Act passed in 1987 guarantees residents the same rights as an individual in the community. The law addresses dignity, self-determination, choice and quality of life. Specifically written and applied to any nursing home receiving Medicare or Medicaid funds it soon became the standard throughout state networks. The law addressed longstanding exploitation and disregard for rights within nursing homes by placing responsibility for human rights directly on the facility. The legislation resulted in a sea change of progress not only for resident's rights but also improved care.
- In 2009 the Affordable Care Act (ACA) began a process of data collection on nursing homes' quality of care and improved transparency in reporting. Resident abuse received considerable attention. With an eye on improved understanding of residents' dementia and decreasing the possibility of abuse, the ACA required dementia and abuse prevention training for staff.
- Most requests considered resident rights are small preferences easily fulfilled. Wishes to differ from the facility routine fall into this category: skip breakfast, no shower today, decline a medication, treatment or therapy session. Nurses record these instances as refusals (refused breakfast, refused shower, etc.). Most instances are not an absolute "No" from the resident, but a simple request. Staff understands such deviations as a resident's right.

- An accumulation of documented refusals in a resident's record will usually be addressed in the care plan as a resident's request and right. An example is skipping breakfast every day resulting in a string of documented refusals. Once a part of the resident's personal care plan she will no longer be expected to go to breakfast.
- When exercising a resident's right becomes a risk to their health and safety, a Release of Responsibility document becomes the nursing home's right. An example is the above resident's right to skip breakfast but later she begins to lose weight.
- One resident's right cannot interfere with another's right. If such conflicts cannot be resolved amicably the nursing home may issue a thirty-day notice of discharge. An example is the resident who refuses showers for weeks on end. His unsanitary presence poses a risk of spreading disease and disagreeable odors among residents and portrays undesirable images for the nursing home.
- Resident-to-resident aggression (RRA) is a serious nursing home issue. Even though resident's rights include the right to be free from harm, altercations, violence and rare homicides occur. Incidents often go unreported and therefore are never investigated. The same interactions seen as intrusions of personal rights in the community cause physical and psychological distress in the nursing home: invasion of privacy and personal space, using personal property without permission, destroying personal property, unwanted sexual behavior, verbal threats and harassment. RRA is considered abuse when one resident willfully harms another. Resident-to–resident abuse is to be reported and investigated as any other abuse.
- In spite of LGBT rights advancement, it remains difficult for residents of long-term care facilities to live openly. Respondents to a recent survey by the National Resource Center on LGBT aging found only twenty-two percent of long-term care residents felt they could be open about sexual identity. Forty-three percent reported mistreatment. Staff training is not mandated and therefore scarce. Advocates point to education as the best route to staff understanding and care of transgender residents.

- Evictions, called involuntary discharges by the industry, increased over the past decade. Targeted residents are usually considered difficult and needing more care or resources. Examples are dementia and severe obesity.
- Sometimes facilities wait until a difficult resident is hospitalized and then deny readmission back into the facility. The usual claim, "We are unable to meet their needs," is easier after a hospital stay.
- There is an appeal process for evictions and refused admission, but the process is slow. Favorable decisions have no teeth or method of enforcement in most cases.
- Each nursing home has a volunteer ombudsman. They are neutral and helpful in resolving disputes between the facility administration and residents, especially resident rights, evictions and refusal to readmit a resident. A call to the ombudsman as soon as problems arise provides the most efficient opportunity for a favorable resolution.
- The facility has a right to reject a resident's request when it conflicts with their organization's philosophy. Although rare, such conflicts do occur. An example would be a resident requesting the right to starve to death. A facility might also refuse to care for a resident with a feeding tube when it conflicts with their stated philosophy. Remember, nursing homes are privately owned business enterprises and their unique exceptions are included in the admission contract.

BEWARE
- Facilities may use a resident's rights claim and release of responsibility document to avoid their own responsibility for reasonable care. An example is the previously mentioned resident who claimed the right to walk without a walker. The nursing home then fails to provide usual help and oversight with walking citing his release of responsibility document even though he has not given up his right to assistance when walking.
- Facilities often extend release of responsibility documents beyond the intended activity. Again, consider the above resident who signed the release of responsibility for walking without a walker. If he falls in the bathroom or trying to get out

of bed because he didn't have needed assistance, the defense for a broken hip will certainly be his release of responsibility document even though he never rejected staff help for walking or any other activity.
- Just before President George W. Bush left office, legal options for neglected or abused nursing home residents were reduced. He signed a bill permitting state inspectors to be treated as federal employees whereby they can be restricted from giving testimony in court. Inspectors identify and track instances of neglect and abuse. Their absence leaves poor treatment of nursing home residents without needed trial evidence.
- Arbitration clauses contained in admission contracts are perhaps the greatest violation of resident's rights. Buried deep in the contracts of 1.5 million nursing home residents are clauses denying the right to court access and a jury trial. A new rule barring arbitration clauses for nursing homes receiving Medicare and Medicaid reimbursement was set to go into effect on November 28, 2016. The industry trade group, The American Health Care Association, successfully blocked the new rule in a Mississippi Court, so arbitration clauses remain in effect today. Additionally, the Trump administration is pushing to scrap the rule completely, thus permitting arbitration clause agreements as a condition of nursing home admission to continue.
- Arbitration clauses move any legal claim against the facility, including wrongful death, into a private system of negotiation influenced and mostly controlled by the nursing home. Courts have upheld arbitration clauses and denied attempts to go around the clauses for a court trial.
- Prior to the ACA crimes against nursing home residents were met with a variety of state regulations. Facility administrators were required to report suspected crimes to the state survey agency, but police involvement was rare. The ACA stipulates that any facility receiving $10,000 in federal funds report any reasonable suspicion of crime against a resident to the state survey agency and local law enforcement.
- Response to a resident's rights issue depends upon the severity of the violation and the resident or their advocate's willingness to pursue a resolution. A matter of inconvenience is best

addressed with the direct care staff. If there is no resolution or if the rights issue is one of safety or neglect you have options: ask for a care plan change, talk with the administrator, call the ombudsman or file a complaint with the state's regulatory agency. Examples include: roommate conflicts, unattended incontinent episodes, missed showers, pain or anxiety resulting from medications delayed or withheld, theft and many others.
- Resident abuse demands immediate attention. If anyone observes abuse, hears of abuse or suspects abuse, an immediate report to staff is crucial because they must protect the victim. Within a few hours follow up with questions: "Was the administrator notified? Was law enforcement notified?" If you receive a report that your loved one has been involved in an abuse incident, the same questions are necessary.
- Observed physical abuse demands an immediate report to law enforcement.

EXAMPLE: How a facility can use a resident's signature on the Release of Responsibility document to justify neglect and attempt protection from legal action.

A fast friendship developed when Mother moved into Loretta's room. Her new roommate was weakened from a stroke, unable to stand and almost bedridden, but delightfully alert. Mother walked about with a walker but needed reminders to use it. She was forgetful, her thinking was muddled and she suffered from an occasional stubborn streak.

Loretta remains an indelible imprint in my mind; always lying flat on her back and rejecting help to turn on her side. The bed's length barely accommodated her lanky six-foot frame. Vibrant blonde locks enhanced by a few silver strands fell below her shoulders as if a flaunting reminder of youthful beauty. She refused haircuts and trims leaving the nursing assistants to style with top of the head ponytails, braids and buns thus no interference with resting her head on the pillow.

Mother seemed to have purpose in helping Loretta with small comforts: a drink of water, finding her tissues, fixing her covers. Loretta became mother's keeper: reminding her to use the walker, shoes for the hallway, a sweater on cold days.

As their friendship developed so did a closeness to each other's family. I expected Loretta to report Mother's transgressions as well as good behavior. She talked with a slow drawl partially because of her stroke but also the influence of her San Antonio heritage. On their weekly visits Loretta's sons received similar updates from Mother. They referred to each other by surnames thus dating their upbringings to a more respectful time. I wondered if there might be a bit of subtle chiding.

"Mrs. Vance was standing in that cold hall last night—nothing on but that flimsy nightgown . . . no walker, no shoes. She didn't turn on her call light, just went looking for pain medicine. I told her to get back in bed and I'd call the nurses. She minds pretty good," typified Loretta's report to me.

Mother's reply, "Well, I can't remember everything. You know, I had to report Mrs. Avery (Loretta) to Edwin (her son) because I caught her trying to eat a big piece of meat that wasn't cut up. Yep, she's impatient too, won't call for help just starts eating."

I chided Mother in front of Loretta, "Don't be ugly to Loretta, you need her. She's the best help you've got."

Loretta beamed and often replied, "Oh, Mrs. Vance is my sister, she helps me more."

Mother remembered little else, but always remembered to check on Loretta's meat. Her stroke left chewing and swallowing problems. The speech therapist recommended ground meat because it was easier to swallow and decreased her risk of choking. Loretta insisted on regular meat, which she could chew and swallow if cut into small bite size pieces. Loretta fed herself but lacked the strength and dexterity needed to cut meat. She signed a Release of Responsibility for her right to be served regular meat. When her meal was served she needed the same help as many fellow residents who needed their meat cut up.

Staff usually served Loretta's meals in her room. Taking her to the dining room was taxing. She required a total lift into the wheelchair—three employees or a mechanical lift and two employees. Transfer to the wheelchair was uncomfortable for Loretta. Her long legs did not fit into any of the facility wheelchairs. Mother took on "Mrs. Avery's meat" as her concern. She always waited to be sure Loretta's meat was cut into bite size pieces before leaving for the dining room and her own meal.

Sometimes a meal with uncut meat was placed in front of Loretta. Mother felt useful in cutting the meat and reporting the staff shortcoming to the nurse in charge. On other occasions she revised staff's cut up meat into smaller pieces to their mutual satisfaction. With Loretta's reminder to "get your walker" she would then be off to the dining room.

After Mother's move to another nursing home my conversation with an employee revealed that Loretta had choked to death on a piece of uncut meat. She was alone in her room. The management's stance, "It was her right to choke to death."

The nursing home's defensive posture neglected their own responsibilities as designated in their license to operate a nursing home. Staff has a basic responsibility for every meal served which is to serve food according to the resident's individual need. The need may be opening packets, arranging silverware or cutting vegetables, bread and meat into edible pieces before walking away. When Loretta was identified as a choking risk by the speech therapist, every meal required constant staff oversight in order to intervene if choking occurred. The nursing home could either assign an employee to stay with her while eating in her room, or take her to the dining room where staff was present to observe for choking. Accordingly, Loretta had the right to sit and eat comfortably in a wheelchair with leg rests long enough to accommodate her physical stature. Loretta did not give up any of these rights by signing a document related to grinding her meat.

I did not mention Loretta's death to Mother. How could I explain the distortion of Loretta's simple rights request into the facility's trivialization of her death?

EXAMPLE: One pathway used to work through a delicate resident's rights issue.

Mr. and Mrs. Hicks occupied the same room for several years. As a new employee, I knocked on their door to announce breakfast. Among Mr. Hick's loud expletives was a demand, "Privacy, privacy!" Nursing assistants rushed to the disturbance. Eyebrows raised, they explained, "We do not open this door between four and eight a.m. Mr. Hicks says, 'That's our private time.'"

Mr. and Mrs. Hicks' request for private time was supported by the social worker's individual conversations with the couple. As Mrs. Hicks became weaker and needed more help with feeding, hygiene and moving out of bed she reinforced her wishes for the private time with her husband. Mr. Hicks needed little assistance and mostly busied himself with oversight of her daily routine: crusty reminders of late linen changes, medications, treatments, etc.

Nursing assistants' occasional grumbles about linen changes and hygiene for Mrs. Hicks after the daily sexual encounters turned to revulsion when Mrs. Hicks became incontinent. They considered exposure to the mixture of body fluids unsafe and asked about HIV and venereal disease testing. Mr. Hicks predictably opened their door at eight a.m. and demanded his wife be cleaned and readied for breakfast. Staff was at their busiest trying to finish the other residents' breakfast, but her hygiene could not be delayed. Odors wafted into the hallway and Mrs. Hicks could not lie in the body fluid mix. Finally, nursing assistants refused to clean the mess.

Nurses agreed with the nursing assistants claiming their right to refuse the cleanup for Mrs. Hicks. Management was nervous; if the couple moved to another nursing home the facility would lose considerable private-pay revenue. The Director of Nursing called a care plan meeting in the couple's room. In attendance were the administrator, social worker, nursing assistants, nurses and housekeeping. The social worker gingerly maneuvered the group to an agreement.

Staff would continue to honor the couples right to early morning privacy. The couple recognized the nursing assistants concern of disagreeable body fluids and the disruption of the other residents breakfast routine. Mr. Hicks agreed to provide his wife hygiene, change the sheets and have Mrs. Hicks ready for breakfast when he opened the door at eight o'clock. Housekeeping would leave clean towels, washcloths and sheets in the room before bedtime each evening along with an empty linen cart for soiled linen.

The arrangement succeeded with the couple maintaining their routine until her death. Mr. Hicks remained a resident until his death.

References

In order to fully appreciate the extent of resident's rights the standards outlined in The Facility Survey Minimum Standards 483.10 is an excellent source.
cms.gov/Medicare/Provider-Enrollment-and-Certification/GuidanceforLawsAndRegulations

ABUSE
New Center for Medicare and Medicaid (CMS) regulations require the staff and administration to report some allegations immediately, i.e., within two hours: abuse, exploitation, neglect, mistreatment, injuries from unknown sources and misappropriation of resident property. If there is no serious injury or no complaint of abuse the reporting period is within twenty-four hours.

RESIDENT-TO-RESIDENT AGGRESSION
CMS State Operations Manual, Guidance to Surveyors for Long Term Care facilities, states that the "facility is responsible for identifying residents who have a history of disruptive or intrusive interactions, or who exhibit other behaviors that make them more likely to be involved in an altercation. The facility should identify the factors (e.g., illness, environment, etc.) that increase the risks associated with individual residents, including those that could trigger an altercation. The care planning team reviews the assessment along with the resident and/or his/her representative, in order to identify interventions to try to prevent altercations."

Aggressive behaviors are often triggered by changes in anti-anxiety and anti-psychotic medication or decreases in dosage.
Resident to Resident Aggression in long-term care facilities: An understudied problem, Aggression and Violent Behavior (2008), doi:10.1016/j.avb.2007.12.001
Deaths as a Result of Resident–to-Resident Altercations in Long-term Care Homes: Editorial, JAMDA 2016.

"The Prevalence of Resident-to-Resident Elder Mistreatment in Nursing Homes (R-REM)," is a study published June 2016 by American College of Physicians. The conclusion: R-REM in nursing homes is highly prevalent. Verbal R-REM is most common, but physical mistreatment also occurs frequently. Because R-REM can cause injury or death, strategies are urgently needed to better understand its causes so that prevention strategies can be developed.

Targeting elder-to-elder mistreatment in long-term care. Results from a cluster randomized trial, International Journal of Nursing Studies (2013), 644-656.

LGBT RIGHTS

The National Resource Center on LGBT Aging—which provides support services to lesbian, gay, bisexual and transgender elders—survey found that respondents were frequently mistreated, including verbal and physical harassment and refused basic services. Some reported being prayed for and warned they might "go to hell" for their sexual orientation and gender identity. Almost ninety percent of LGBT residents predicted that staff members would discriminate based on unspoken homophobia.

Staying Out Of The Closet in Old Age, Anna Gorman, Kaiser Health News, October 17, 2016

ARBITRATION CLAUSES

Judge Michael Mills, U.S. District Court of the Northern District of Mississippi: "Congress' failure to enact positive legislation should not serve as an excuse for the executive branch to assume powers which are properly reserved for the legislative branch."

Vermont Senator Patrick Leahy: "The sad reality is that today too many Americans must choose between forfeiting legal rights and getting adequate medical care." Senator Leahy refers to the clauses now forcing arbitration in almost all nursing home admission contracts.

The nursing home industry, represented by their trade organization, The American Health Care Association says arbitration is less costly than court. They speak of lawsuits driving up costs and forcing facilities to close.

Resident advocates note residents enter nursing homes at a stressful time in their life. They need the care and do not fully grasp what they are signing. Even if they understand they are hard pressed to find a facility without the arbitration clause. Arbitration proceedings are confidential and information is never collected for nursing home databases. Corporate ownership is able to keep disturbing neglect and liability from public scrutiny. Awards in arbitration hearings are far less than jury trials.

Lawyers representing the elderly have been unable to overturn arbitration clauses. In one case, a man who could not read or write signed his name to a nursing home contract containing an arbitration clause. The appeals court reasoned, "illiteracy alone is not a sufficient basis for the invalidation of an arbitration agreement."

Trump Moves to Impede Consumer Lawsuits Against Nursing Homes, Robert Pear, *The New York Times*, August 18, 2017.

EVICTIONS
Medicaid beneficiaries comprise the majority of involuntary discharges. The most vulnerable Medicaid residents are those on the low end of the Medicaid reimbursement scale. Facilities prefer to fill beds with Medicare rehabilitation and private-pay residents whom they consider more profitable than long-term Medicaid residents.

Private-pay residents become vulnerable to evictions when private funds are exhausted and the resident becomes a Medicaid beneficiary.

"As Nursing Homes Evict Patients," States Question Motives, Ina Jaffe, *NPR*, May 26, 2017.

RESOURCES
National Long-Term Care Ombudsman Resource Center (NORC)
    Elder Abuse/Elder Justice Issue page (includes resident-to-resident) mistreatment fact sheet
    http://ltcombudsman.org/issues
National Center for Elder Abuse (NCEA)
    Elder abuse, neglect or exploitation
    https://ncea.acl.gov/ or call 855-500-3537

Kaiser Health News, "Rising Obesity Puts Strain on Nursing Homes," Sarah Varney, December 15, 2015

RESIDENT'S RIGHTS
Your Rights and Protections as a Nursing Home Resident

"What are my rights in a nursing home? As a nursing home resident, you have certain rights and protections under Federal and state law that help ensure you get the care and services you need. You have the right to be informed, make your own decisions, and have your personal information kept private.

"The nursing home must tell you about these rights and explain them in writing in a language you understand. They must also explain in writing how you should act and what you're responsible for while you're in the nursing home. This must be done before or at the time you're admitted, as well as during your stay. You must acknowledge in writing that you got this information."
cms.gov/medicare/Your_Resident_Rights_and_Protections_section

CHAPTER 11

MEDICATIONS

Medications play a significant role in the operation of nursing homes and their residents' lives. Facilities have the duty and expense of securing, storing and getting medications to their residents. Licensed nurses are a critical link. They communicate with physicians and pharmacists, schedule medications and assure that they are given at the right time. In addition, nurses' education, training and experience are vital components in evaluating medication effects (desired versus undesirable results).

For residents and their families there is the selection of a pharmacy, medication expenses and an awareness of how each medication affects themselves or their loved one. We are all familiar with drug warnings and precautions. Each drug category from antibiotics to water pills comes with potential problems: nausea, fatigue, diarrhea, etc. Still, we accept the necessity of medications for treatment of diseases and symptoms. Drugs often provide comfort. The observations of the resident, family and friends are important as nurses and physicians adjust medications.

Medicines considered as mind or mood altering carry additional responsibility for the facility and the resident. This collection of drugs treats depression, sleeplessness, anxiety, confusion, psychotic disorders, disturbing behaviors, pain or even the perception that any of these conditions exist. Controversy abounds over the use of these medications. Reports of over-sedated, drooling residents slumped in wheelchairs is countered by reports of agitated, yelling residents thought to need sedation. Both situations violate residents' rights; the first to be free of chemical restraints (drugs), and the second to be free of pain whether mental or physical.

Many residents are alert and comfortable because of mood altering medications. Nevertheless, barriers to managing these drugs in nursing homes often seem insurmountable. Most mood-altering medicines are controlled substances. Nursing homes' accountability for storing and dispensing these medications contribute to facility anxieties and tedious procedures involving each dose of each drug.

Residents caught in this conundrum often receive the least of considerations even though observations and symptoms support a resident's need for their medication.

Mood-altering medications may be ordered when they are *not* needed. Better staffing, consistent caregiver assignments, varied activities and improved training may be sufficient, but these are management decisions. Residents and their families are left to work within facility limitations. Best results are obtained when responsible parties, families and residents state clear expectations to physicians and nursing home staff, then persist with oversight and advocacy. It is reasonable to expect that your loved one will attain a stable mood and maintain their mental alertness and physical agility.

The BE AWARE and BEWARE sections offer help in understanding and navigating through your loved one's medications. EXAMPLES include institutional failures and successful communication with a physician.

BE AWARE
- If a patient is admitted for skilled nursing care under Medicare Part A, prescriptions will generally be covered by Part A. When Medicare Part A coverage ends the resident becomes responsible for medication charges.
- The nursing home keeps a few medications on hand for emergency situations. Residents' regular medications are ordered from outside pharmacies using individual payment sources: Medicare D, Medicaid, insurance or private pay.
- You may continue using your local pharmacy even though the nursing home will steer you toward their contracted pharmacy services. That contract will be with one of the national pharmaceutical chains often located in distant cities.
- During patient transfers from hospitals to nursing homes, medications ordered from remote pharmacies may not be delivered for twenty-four hours or longer. It is important to coordinate the availability of critical drugs, especially pain medication, to assure medications are on hand soon after the new resident's admission.
- Medicare does not tell physicians which medications to order even though pharmacy and facility often promote this idea. Sometimes a resident's insurance plan denies payment for a

specific drug, but more often the nursing home's contracted pharmacy service does not have the medication available. For example, a resident using the facility's contracted pharmacy is told, "Medicare won't pay for this drug." If the contracted pharmacy's formulary (the list of medications available from their company) does not include the medication, it is easier to blame Medicare than search for the medication at competing pharmacies.
- Participation in your loved one's overall medication regimen is an endless chore. However, mood-altering medications require closer oversight for changes in drugs, dosage and scheduling, in order to maximize benefit and minimize undesired effects.
- There are safeguards against the excessive use of mood-altering medications or even using them when they are *not* needed; protections include state inspections, data collection discouraging use, pharmacy reviews and your observations. Communication with the physician who orders the medication is essential. The resident or responsible party stating their expectations is a helpful guide as the physician changes medications and adjusts dosage.
- Essential questions to the physician ordering a medication and the other professionals involved in your loved one's care include: (1) Why is the medication being ordered? (2) What is the intended result—sleeping better at night, less worry and crying, stopping hallucinations, fewer emotional outbursts? (3) How soon are results expected, a few days or maybe weeks? (4) What side effects should we look for—drowsiness, loss of appetite, weight gain?
- Mood-altering medications used to treat the symptoms of anxiety disorders, psychoses and pain fall into a broad category of drugs designated as controlled substances by the Federal Drug Administration. Federal regulations and sometimes, additional state rules impact how these drugs are ordered and dispensed to residents.
- Nursing homes develop controlled substance routines to comply with drug laws and data collection for government agencies and inspectors. For the facility, residents' medication needs are less important than following these procedures.

BEWARE

Many nursing home policies complicate a resident's access to mood-altering drugs.

- Data is collected on the number of mood-altering medications dispensed in each nursing home. Increased numbers or percentages are perceived to increase regulatory scrutiny therefore the focus is largely on decreasing the use of these medications.
- If a resident is *not* experiencing undesired side effects, meddling with a medication regimen to protect the facility's statistics is unacceptable.
- A registered pharmacist reviews each resident's entire medication regimen at least monthly. The purpose is to assure that all medications are ordered and given correctly. During these reviews the pharmacist pays particular attention to mood-altering medications because they are considered chemical restraints. Therefore, according to industry mindset, attempts to reduce the dosage or eliminate the drug verify the facility's good faith effort to reduce restraints.
- The pharmacist, a facility paid consultant, routinely recommends dosage decreases or changes in mood-altering medications during reviews. The pharmacist's recommendations are based on behavioral data and medication records collected by the nursing staff. Often there is more nursing information missing than is present. A resident's instability created by pharmacist's recommended medication changes is rarely a consideration.
- Mood-altering medication changes are usually proposed as a trial with the idea that you can return to the original dose if the resident deteriorates. Some residents never recover.
- Pharmacist's recommendations are sent to the attending physician for review and approval. Usually the pharmacist's suggestions are authorized because physicians depend upon the facility's routine for compliance with controlled substance laws. Physicians who receive patient referrals from the facility are unlikely to disagree with the facility's pharmacist.

- Nurses often ask physicians to discontinue medications they have not used for a while. Such requests may just be nurses wanting to clean out their medicine drawer, simplify their medication sheets or cut the time needed to count controlled medicines between shifts. Nurses' tidiness also supports their idea that decreasing the number of controlled drugs on hand, decreases the number of questions and the possibility of problems from inspectors. If the resident needs the same medication again it is treated as a new drug and the order process begins anew: call physician for order, contact pharmacy, wait for delivery and a new medication cost.

National and regional contracts impact individual resident's care.
- Nursing home corporations contract with pharmaceutical corporations for all pharmacy services within the building. Included is a pharmacist who reviews the residents' medication regimen monthly. Most of the facility residents' medications are ordered through the contracted pharmacy, therefore a lucrative revenue source for the pharmacy company. Sometimes the contracted pharmacy is a separate holding of the nursing home chain. Many contractual agreements are nationwide and will always take precedence over a resident's wellbeing.
- If a medication is changed or the dosage decreased, a new medication will be ordered and the old medication destroyed. Even if the old medication is restarted a few days later, a completely new prescription will be issued by the pharmacy, thus a new charge to Medicare, Medicaid or you.

Nurses give mood-altering drugs on two different timetables.
- Some medicines are given on a regular schedule. Others are given when a specific need arises such as pain and anxiety.
- A doctor may order a regularly scheduled medication with additional doses to be given at nurses' discretion, for reasons such as resident anxious, pacing, uncontrolled pain.
- Desired schedules are those which move toward regular, routine medications; stabilizing the resident's mood, and therefore, gradually decreasing the need for extra medications or the as needed drugs.

- The resident or their agent's (responsible party) signed consent must be obtained prior to beginning many of these drugs.
- Prior to decreasing dosage or stopping a medicine, consent is *not* required.

Staffing affects resident's medications.
- Use of mood-altering medications as chemical restraints occurs more often in facilities with inadequate direct care staff.
- Caregivers are often untrained in the complexities of mood-altering medications and ill prepared to administer them properly or identify desirable or undesirable effects.
- Unfamiliar faces of temporary staffing and new staff members often trigger apprehension in residents, thus increased need for medications.
- New staff cannot be expected to identify mood swings or behaviors needing medication. Regular staff becomes familiar with each resident's idiosyncrasies; therefore, they are more likely to recognize changes, provide alternative interventions or administer medication before a crisis develops.

There are methods of ensuring that your resident receives the best medication regimen.
- Your best hope of stability is oversight of mood-altering medications by a psychiatrist or gerontologist.
- Establish a definite understanding of your wishes with the attending physician. Can you accept, for example, some drowsiness in exchange for anxiety relief?
- Putting your wishes in writing for the physician will serve as a reminder when problems occur. Such documentation will also serve as legal cover for the physician and offer a rebuttal to nursing home requests for changes. Be sure to sign all written communication.
- Develop an efficient method of communication with the physician whether email, texting or fax. Phone calls are an *inefficient* use of a physician's time. They frequently involve delays for return calls or may go unanswered. Messages left with office staff rarely remain intact when relayed to the doctor.
- Get the social worker involved. Most are familiar with mood-altering medications. They have more time for discussion and

can facilitate communication between family, staff and physicians.
- Seek out and become acquainted with a caring nurse or nursing assistant on each shift. After gaining their trust this handful of special employees will give dependable reports and take interest in your resident's wellbeing when you are not there.
- Make your wishes and expectations known in care plan meetings.
- Instruct in writing that mood-altering medications are not to be changed (increased or decreased) without contacting the responsible party first. Ask that these instructions be placed in a prominent place in the resident's medical record.
- Physicians can place a statement in the resident's chart giving a reason for indefinite use of a medication and thus sidestep the pharmacist's recommendations of decreasing dosage and changing medications. Few physicians know of this option and when informed may hesitate to use it, citing litigation potential. The resident once again becomes a secondary concern.

Be suspicious of nursing home employees who tell you, "The State (inspectors) tells us we have to decrease mind-altering meds."
- Inspector's focus is residents' well-being.
- Inspectors will not compromise residents well-being by questioning a medication regimen when professionals fulfill their responsibility.
- Professional responsibility includes: (1) A signed doctor's order giving a reason not to change medications. (2) A care plan in place for medications not to be changed. (3) A directive for the facility to call the responsible party prior to any medication change.

Medications specific to the treatment of psychoses require frequent evaluation and adjustment. The resident's condition and good medical practice should guide decisions, not facility statistics.

EXAMPLE: How institutional drug reviews and procedures become more important than a resident's wellbeing.

MEDICATIONS

Maggie exhibited unusual amiability considering her psychiatric history and current residency, the secure unit within a San Antonio nursing home. Unlike her peers, Maggie never spoke of escaping the locked doors instead she chose to become completely engaged in the unit's confined activities. Occasionally, staff escorted Maggie to gatherings with the regular nursing home residents. She enjoyed musical presentations and sing-alongs. A master of pleasant conversation and etiquette she often engaged residents, staff and visitors.

Maggie was devoted to her personal appearance and managed an impressive wardrobe. She wore skirts and dresses of finely woven fabric, no pants, slacks or denims. No sport shoes or sandals, she chose slight heels with matching accessories. Her sinewy six-foot frame never appeared outside her room until adorned in her elegant style. Her ensembles captured the rainbow's mystique, but as individual colors: blue, pink, yellow green, lilac and white. None matched the richness of her ebony skin.

Maggie's medication schedule was just as impressive. It included multiple mind-altering medications with maximum dosage and dire warnings of possible bad effects. Her psychiatrist worked with family and staff for months fine-tuning the regimen.

After years of erratic behavior and psychiatric hospitalizations her son voiced pride in his mother's stable mood. She swayed on his arm as he escorted her to church every Sunday morning. Maggie always reminded the nurse, "Don't save my lunch, I'll be eating out."

I received a Saturday morning report of Maggie's explosion but it took a walk into the secure unit to understand the seriousness. Entry revealed chaos. Wall hangings and pictures were askew or missing. The corridor was abandoned, a stark contradiction to the breakfast hour's usual business of food, linen and housekeeping carts. Doors to residents' rooms were shut. There were no residents, visitors or staff in sight.

Two additional hallways branching from the nurse's station were also deserted except for Maggie. She was squared off in her room's doorway: one foot in her room, one foot in the hallway, a hand on her hip and the other atop the doorway's header. She stared stone-faced at the nurses in bold defiance. Her disheveled appearance defined her personal angst. Standing barefoot, one strap of her fine silk slip off shoulder left the hem dragging low on one side. Maggie wore no other attire, not even dentures.

Despondent nurses explained the routine procedures leading to Maggie's distress. On his monthly review, the pharmacist recommended a dosage decrease in one medication—he was concerned about inspector citations for chemical restraints. Her physician was off-duty and his physician's assistant ordered the change even though a nurse questioned it.

Within twenty-four hours Maggie became suspicious of staff, refused any medication, then progressed to violent behavior. They pointed to the broken chair, torn drapes and uprooted plant stacked in the corner.

Her favorite nurse said, "Maggie stripped her closets and room of everything not anchored. She threw the lot on the beds, threatened her roommate and used the furniture to barricade herself in the room. Her son is so worried."

The charge nurse asked, "Why did they mess with Maggie's medicine? She hasn't slept for forty-eight hours. Everybody worked on a transfer yesterday afternoon but the psychiatric hospitals won't accept her until they can come check, of course that means Monday. Ambulances won't transfer her to the emergency room—said 'we're not trained for violent patients.'"

We faced the worst of circumstances on this Saturday morning. Preventing Maggie from escalating into rages required planning. The potential for such fury causing physical injury to herself, fellow residents and staff dominated our thoughts. The strong injection her physician ordered to calm her must be given every four hours. Giving the painful shot required physical restraint by four staff members thus increasing the risk of injury to both Maggie and her nurses.

Monday did not bring relief for Maggie or her family. She was transferred to a psychiatric hospital; her paranoid behavior continued; she was finally placed in a high security facility known for warehousing people.

Maggie was the victim of institutional routine geared to protect the nursing home from inspectors' scrutiny. Specifically, the pharmacist fulfilled his contractual obligation for the pharmaceutical company and the physician's assistant efficiently followed his recommendations. A simple call to Maggie's son prior to medication changes and a physician's documentation of indefinite need provided the best deterrent to her disaster. Staff had not offered her son or the physician the options.

EXAMPLE: Harm caused by an institutional pharmacy review and a new nurse, unfamiliar with the residents.

"Mrs. Lovett?"
"Yes."
"Mrs. Vance asked me to call you." *Oh no! A 7:00 am, Sunday phone call from the nursing home means trouble.*
"Okay, that's good," I replied. *This is a new nurse—proper names, professional tone, the regular nurses would have diverted Mother to breakfast.*
Mother pleaded through sobs. "Oh, honey, please help me. I can't find George. He's looking for me. He can't find me. He's worried about me. Please try to find him. Tell him I'm okay. Oh honey, I need help."
"Mother, I'll be right there. Let me speak to the nurse." I asked several times as her repetitions accelerated. She was distraught when the nurse returned to the phone.
"Please give Mother her anti-anxiety pill and I will be right there." *How could any nurse not see that she needs medication.*
The nurse said, "Looks like she hadn't needed it for a while so the pharmacist recommended it be stopped a few days ago."
I thought; *How can this happen? There are instructions in Mother's chart to notify me before any medication changes.* "Please give her pain medication."
"But she's not complaining of pain," the nurse said.
"Well, mother has dementia and she usually can't verbalize her pain. When she becomes restless, starts pacing and mumbling we know she's in pain. If she doesn't get pain relief she becomes anxious, but I've never seen her like this. Please check her left knee. I think you'll find it tender, red and swollen. Mother really needs her pain medicine and I'm on my way."
I fought back tears as I entered the nursing home. Mother sat alone on the entryway bench, bundled in her favorite fleece jacket. She seemed to be seeking her own comfort; with crossed arms she hugged her chest, slouched forward and shivered. *How could any resident be left alone in such a painful, emotional crisis?* Her white athletic shoes and bulky, neon yellow socks contrasted sharply with her

demure black slacks but assured me she was feeling feisty when she dressed this morning. Aromas and sounds of breakfast wafted from the dining room.

"Oh Honey, thank God you're here, thank God you're here," she sobbed and trembled through a high-pitched voice. Mother called me "Honey" when she couldn't remember my name . . . another indication of her stress level. "Honey, George is looking for me. He can't find me. He's so worried."

"Mother, now remember, Daddy's been gone for a while." *Actually, forty-five years.*

"I know that but he's looking for me."

"Mother, Daddy's just fine. He wants us to take care of you."

"Well, what am I supposed to do?" She threw her arms open, tears cascaded.

"Just sit here. I'm gonna get us some coffee."

"Honey, just cool mine with a little bit of water?"

"Mother, let's go to my house and I'll make us some good coffee?"

"No. I'm gonna sit right here so George can find me." Crying ceased, but she remained on high alert—eyes wide open, eyebrows raised, forehead furrowed. Her red swollen face strained to see who might be entering the building.

"Mother, don't move. You don't have your walker. I don't want you to fall and break a leg. You've got enough trouble already."

"Well, so what? They could just shoot me while I'm down. Ain't that what they do to horses?" Her *characteristic sassiness is replacing the anxiety.*

My sprint to the nurse's station located her walker beside the phone she used. *Why wouldn't somebody assist her with the walker, especially since she's identified as a fall risk?*

The nurse confirmed giving her pain medication. *There is no benefit to making an issue of Mother's anxiety medicine with her—an out of town agency nurse . . . never worked here before . . . will never work here again. Besides, I can't leave Mother without her walker; she's already forgotten my instructions not to get up if it ever registered in the first place.* I planted the walker in front of Mother and hurried for coffee.

"Honey, did you water that down?"

"No Mother, I did not water it down. You said just a little water to cool it down and that's what I did."

"Don't get ugly with me! I guess that woman sure thinks she's something." Mother referenced a churchgoer in her Sunday best entering the door. *Oh no! I hope the lady didn't hear.*

A decreasing anxiety level indicated Mother simply needed diversion and companionship to avoid another frenzy. A blank Sunday activity schedule relegated us to the bench and conversation. Additional residents joined us. Lively conversation circled through the cluster: greeting visitors, critiquing their attire and identifying each with a particular resident. Two ladies with deep community roots added details of divorces, bankruptcies and infidelities.

I stayed until after lunch, helped Mother to bed for a nap and depended on her bedfast, but alert and protective roommate to call me if needed. A good nurse was scheduled to come on duty at 3:00 pm. The medication mess must wait until tomorrow when management personnel return to work.

Mother's experience provides an example of the persistence required to overcome task oriented, institutional priorities. Such mindset easily ignores individual resident conditions, doctor's orders and family requests. Do not expect anyone in management to acknowledge the emotional upset and pain suffered by the resident nor the family's frustration, lost time and resources spent correcting each situation.

EXAMPLE: A communication letter attempting to clarify medication expectations. The previous night, Mother complained of chest pain, the facility called an ambulance and sent her to the emergency room. Several weeks previously her medication had been decreased after a routine pharmacy review.

Dear Dr. _____

Re: Ola Bell Vance

>At mother's last care plan meeting we discussed the decrease of Mother's Ativan to prn only. Nursing administration agreed they would have staff chart any symptoms of stress or anxiety. Within the last 2-3 weeks. I've observed more worry and restlessness in

the evening hours. Her worry is concentrated on getting back to Powell—her old home in Wyoming.

If I'm not there by shortly after supper she is calling me with the same question. Don't mind the call, but she just can't wait until I get there. I've asked the evening nurses to document this for your review, but they tell me they don't usually document resident requests to make phone calls, they can usually redirect her and they can give the Ativan when needed.

They are very kind and caring. However, my thoughts are that she should not be worried in the first place. I believe the extent of her worry is emotionally painful to her. Sometimes agency nurses are there who really can't be expected to differentiate her baseline emotional state. My vote is to return to the regular afternoon/evening dose of Ativan. I visit her almost every day—usually after supper because she doesn't remember I've been there if I come before supper.

I never found her to be sedated or drowsy with the old med regimen. She is still doing great during the day. I think her symptoms last night started with the same worry, I didn't go to see her last evening and she just worked herself into a dither.

Sincerely,

Frances Lovett

Mother's physician faxed a copy of the letter to the nursing home with an order to return to her previous schedule of giving Ativan each evening on a regular basis.

References

PUBLIC OPINION: The public outcry and much publicized photos of stuporous, drooling residents slumped in wheelchairs was the beginning of current oversight of mood-altering medications as chemical restraints.

OVERSIGHT: Data collected on admission and at regular intervals is transmitted to state and federal databases tied to each facility's provider number. Statistics compiled from the general population of each nursing home is posted on the federal website. Facilities do not want to be associated with a large percentage of their residents receiving mood-altering medications. When inspectors/surveyors enter the facility they have a computer printout of all residents on these medications. They will target these residents for review.

The accepted practice is to decrease the number of medications or dosage (strength and frequency) amount about every three months. Theoretically, in doing so, the facility shows a good faith effort toward reducing chemical restraints and decreases the risk of associated citations and deficiencies.

BEHAVIORS: Consumers should ask nursing homes about their approach to managing behavior. Interventions that don't require medications, like higher staffing ratios, many and varied activities, and consistent assignment, have been shown to be successful in many cases. gov/nursinghomecompare/search.html (search: staffing: long stay residents who got antipsychotic medications)

Misuse of Antipsychotic Drugs—chemical restraints and abuse: "There is a solution to this form of elder abuse! Improve staffing levels in nursing facilities. Long-standing evidence confirms that nursing facilities employ too few nurses to meet residents' needs." Center for Medicare Advocacy: "Elder Abuse in Nursing Facilities: The Over-Administration of Antipsychotic Drugs to Nursing Home Residents:"

Detrimental effects of inadequate and poorly trained staff are plentiful. *The Primer for Managed Care Organizations* (p. 36) provides a concise overview. " . . . inappropriate antipsychotic drug use is often associated with systemic problems in a facility, such as insufficient staffing and a lack of knowledge and/or use of nonpharmacological

treatment options for dementia care.
http://www.ltccc.org/publications/documents/LTCCC-Primer-Nursing-Home-Quality-for-MCO-FINAL_000.pdf

CHAPTER 12

MEALTIME

The impact of mealtime on residents' wellbeing cannot be overstated. Indeed, meals separate good nursing homes from bad nursing homes. Three times a day good facilities serve each resident nutritious, appetizing food, assure enough staff to assist with eating and do so in a stimulating environment.

Recalling our own hunger or thirst during delays in meals or fluids lends understanding to the discomfort residents suffer during bad mealtimes. One occurrence leaves the resident hungry and weak. Repeated episodes have cumulative health effects, such as dehydration, malnutrition and pain.

Residents eat in either a community dining room or their individual rooms. The dining room is a therapeutic experience, encompassing the benefits of nutrition, exercise and social interaction. The gathering also provides the staff with an efficient opportunity to observe multiple residents for individual changes in mental status and physical abilities.

Eating in the dining room is impossible for some. Infections, fractures with traction, open wounds and complex medical care are a few examples. Residents have a right to eat in their own rooms, but the practice is discouraged because it leaves them secluded.

A mealtime visit offers insight into the overall tenor of a facility. Is the dining room vibrant, active and alive with interaction between staff and residents? Is it dull and morose? Why are there empty chairs? Are the absentees left isolated in their rooms because of short staffing or lax supervision?

Dining room meals may seem chaotic even when they are going well. However, your own observations and good judgment allow you to separate the good from the bad. Is everyone eating? Do residents have the help they need? No one should be sitting unattended if food remains on his/her plate. Some need to be spoon-fed, others eat independently, but need a word of encouragement to take the last few bites. A resident may lack the energy to finish eating and needs to be spoon-fed the remainder.

Residents eating in their rooms need the same personal attention, but in facilities lacking adequate nursing staff, they may not receive the care.

Mealtimes trigger a shutdown of all other resident centered activities. The all-hands-on-deck effort coordinates responsibilities of nursing, dietary and housekeeping staffs. They must get residents to the dining room, prepare and serve each a meal and assure that it is eaten. Then the labor of returning residents to their rooms and cleaning up the dining room mess begins.

The BE AWARE and BEWARE sections are a guide to expectations for your loved one's meals. The EXAMPLE walks the reader through one dining room experience. APPENDIX C is a deeper dive into facility responsibilities.

BE AWARE
- Residents need different levels of assistance to get dressed and into the dining room. Expect your loved one to receive all the help they need to get to their assigned table on time.
- Tables are usually arranged to seat four residents. It is important for your loved one to sit with residents having similar physical and mental capacities.
- Expect your loved one to be seated with a group having similar diets. It can be impossible to explain why one resident receives a fruit cup for desert and another lemon merengue pie, especially to a confused resident perceiving they are being treated differently.
- Mealtimes are an opportunity for pleasurable experiences especially when favorite foods are served. Desserts often gain the earliest attention and your loved one has a right to eat it first.
- Added assurance that each resident eats well is to avoid serving them foods they dislike. The kitchen has a list of foods your loved one won't eat and you can expect a substitute of equal nutritional value when these foods are on the menu.
- Personal menus and food selection has become a marketing strategy for some facilities.
- Person-centered care directives issued by the Centers for Medicare and Medicaid Services (CMS) in November of 2016 and consumer advocacy are moving nursing homes toward

individual menu selections. Meaningful choices reflecting religious, cultural and ethnic preferences are woven into the new guidelines. However, the new administration issued guidelines placing the directives on hold for 2018.
- Each nursing home has a contractual agreement with a nutritionist (Registered Dietitian or RD), who oversees the facility's monthly menu. This menu assures that each day's meal plan provides a balanced diet with adequate nutrition and fluids when it is followed.
- Expect all the residents at a table to be served their meal at the same time. Most of us would consider it cruel for anyone at the table to be without food while others are eating.
- Nursing home standards require hot foods to be served hot and cold foods cold.
- When a resident's meal arrives, staff is expected to set it up completely before leaving. A few residents need a little help, maybe opening packets. Others need more help: arranging silverware, placing cups and glasses within easy reach, cutting meat into bite size pieces and buttering bread or the stimulation of feeding them their first bite.
- Sometimes residents don't feel well or for unknown reasons reject the meal they are served. There is always an alternative meal on the menu; it should be offered when this happens. A peanut butter and jelly sandwich is not an acceptable alternative.
- If your loved one needs to be spoon fed their meal should *not* be placed in front of them until someone is available to assist.
- Residents who need total assistance with eating may be seated at a crescent shaped table, sometimes called a feeder table. One nurse's aide sits inside the C shape and feeds residents seated around the outside. The arrangement allows one nurse's aide to feed more than one resident, but they should not attempt to feed more than three residents at a time. Again, all residents sitting together should have the same mental awareness.
- A few nursing homes serve family style meals at selective tables for residents able to serve and feed themselves. These arrangements still require constant oversight by a nurse or nurse's aide.

- Nursing home standards require the same attention and assistance be given to residents eating in their rooms as those eating in the dining room. Even those who eat without assistance need to be checked at intervals. Rarely is there enough staff for this one-on-one care in residents' rooms, whereas the dining room allows one staff member to oversee numerous residents.
- Minimum standards require the presence of a licensed nurse (RN, LVN, LPN) in the dining room from the time the first resident is served until the last resident finishes eating.

BEWARE
- Regulations require the facility to provide each resident three regular meals daily in accordance to normal mealtimes. Most facilities schedule meals at 7 a.m., 12 noon and 5 p.m. There can be no more than fourteen hours between the evening meal and breakfast. If a nourishing snack is served at bedtime up to sixteen hours is allowed between the evening meal and breakfast. Few nursing homes provide bedtime snacks without a specific doctor's order.
- There is a considerable difference in serving each resident something to eat at bedtime and the usual practice of simply having a few snacks available on the nursing units for residents who are able to make a request.
- Mealtime may be the only time residents are offered liquids so it is important for each one to drink as much as possible during meals. The RD has calculated how many ounces each resident should drink with meals especially those who are on restricted fluids.
- Special diets are often simplified because of kitchen limitations. Preparing complicated diets is time consuming and expensive. They are frequently prepared incorrectly because of kitchen staff's limited training and therefore become a source of deficiencies during inspections. Examples: a calculated diabetic regimen may be changed to "no concentrated sweets" or a strict sodium restriction to "no added salt".
- Each facility has an employee responsible for the kitchen operations. They are usually called the Food Service Director (FSD) or something similar. This person receives training in

managing food preparation and kitchen operations. They are helpful in resolving food likes and dislikes for your resident and complaints about food service. An FSD lacks the knowledge needed to advise in serious nutritional problems such as malnutrition and electrolyte imbalances.
- The RD is usually a contract person and spends limited time in the facility. They oversee the menu, advise the FSD on state inspection standards and check on residents with weight loss or nutritional problems. RDs are a great asset to physicians, nurses and residents faced with difficult dietary problems. Their education includes advanced degrees. They hold a state licensure. The RD is available to evaluate your loved one's nutritional status if you have concerns. There is no additional charge for the consult.
- If your loved one is losing weight here are key questions to ask: Are they eating all their food at mealtime? Do they need more physical help to eat? Are they too tired to eat after sitting and waiting too long for their meal?
- A practice to watch for is decreased size of regular servings. Examples would be cutting vegetable servings from one-half cup to a fourth-cup, decreasing meat servings from four ounces to two ounces or serving a half sandwich instead of the whole sandwich. Unscrupulous nursing homes use this tactic to save money on food. It is most often seen at the evening meal where there are fewer visitors and less scrutiny.
- Lack of dental care and ill-fitting dentures often interfere with a resident's ability to eat. Even though soft foods and ground meat can be served, eating is still painful when dental care is needed.
- The current month's daily menu calendar should be posted in the dining room. If a facility does not serve meals according to this schedule it probably indicates they are cutting corners on their food budget. Certainly residents are not being fed according to the Registered Dietician's nutritional calculations. Therefore, the nursing home is violating their state license to operate a nursing home.

EXAMPLE: This overview of an average mealtime captures the camaraderie of staff and residents, the old and young and varied backgrounds.

The nursing home dining room was in full bloom. I circulated around the small tables, each seated two to four residents. Clinking silverware and dishes, fragrant cabbage, a big spill, clanking pots in the kitchen and flourishing conversations contributed to the colorful chaos.

I overheard a nurse's aide, "Mr. Garcia, open your eyes, let's eat."

"Why? You gonna poke it in my eyes?" he asked.

Overheard from another table, "Papa, you cleaned that pie up plenty fast. Now try the rest of your food. The mashed potatoes are real good."

"Well, I'd like to git'n that kitchen and show 'em how to mash potatoes," a plump lady groused before finishing her last bite.

"Not me, Oma. I've mashed the last potato I intend to in this lifetime," came a screeching response from across the table.

A nurse's aide yelled, "Somebody help Jake with his turkey."

As I moved through the dining room I noticed a thin, muscular man who wasn't eating. His full white Afro drew attention to his deep facial wrinkles. He stared out the window, detached from his lunch. The other residents at the table were finished.

I said, "Mr. Lee, aren't you hungry? Would you like something different to eat?" The question elicited nothing more than a sad stare in my direction.

"Does he usually eat?" I asked a nearby nurse's aide.

"He's not acting right," she answered. "I tried to feed him, but he just shuts his mouth. They moved him out of the locked unit last week and he misses his friends in there." I wrote, "refused" on his diet report and made a mental note to check on him later.

I moved across the room to check on a spastic black arm waving for attention. Mr. Allen, the middle-aged resident couldn't talk, but he indicated with a downward thrust of his arm that Mrs. Giles needed help. The aged, frail lady sat across the table. She was unable to speak.

Mr. Allen's right side was paralyzed forcing him into an unnatural wheelchair posture. His stiff leg protruded forward from a hip and knee joint that would not bend to accommodate sitting. His elbow and shoulder were frozen anchoring his arm tightly against his chest. Mr. Allen's right hand was fixed forever beneath his chin.

His left forefinger gestured forcefully and repeatedly from his coffee toward Mrs. Giles. We were both frustrated by the time I understood he was asking me to get her some coffee, then no cream and then no sugar and finally, just black. Each response elicited jerks and forward thrusts of his entire body. His neck veins became engorged and his facial muscles tightened. After several missed signals, I finally interpreted his grunts as "yes" and his squeals as "no."

Mrs. Giles sat motionless.

I warned her, "It's very hot, please be careful." Mr. Allen became anxious again. He pointed to his own iced tea to help me understand she needed ice to cool it down. I retrieved ice chips and got the measurement down to the half-teaspoon he thought the situation required. He smiled, attempted to say "thank you" but settled for a gentle wave of his hand.

I said, "Thank you, Mr. Allen, I appreciate your help."

Mrs. Giles remained indifferent to the turmoil surrounding her coffee. A young nurse's aide slipped behind the table, raised her eyebrows, smiled and gave an understanding nod.

I waited to be sure Mrs. Giles could manage her coffee and recognized her mannerisms to be those of a sophisticated lady. She sat upright, aloof to her surroundings and took only small bites and sips. Her napkin was ever present. A dainty white face hinted of fine porcelain. It was framed perfectly by the silver strands of hair escaping her bun, which had gone askew. Her batiste blouse was embellished with soft pastel threads and a delicate, ruffled collar reminiscent of an earlier era.

Mr. Allen's trendy knit shirt sporting a Cowboys logo placed him squarely in the current decade. Staff must have struggled to pull the shirt over his contorted arm and attend to the details of his meticulous grooming.

I circulated back to Mr. Lee's table. A young Latino nurse's aide was feeding him the last few bites. The nurse's aide I talked with earlier said, "I called Raul for help. He works in the locked unit and Papa knows and trusts him." Papa is the respectful term of endearment afforded elderly gentlemen in South Texas.

I said, "Thank you for your help Raul."

"Don't need thanks Ma'am. Papa's my friend," Raul did not move his eyes from the task at hand. The twinkle in Mr. Lee's eyes confirmed the friendship.

Well, let me change that diet report to ate one hundred per cent.

Most residents had finished eating and the slow trip back to their rooms was underway. I spotted Mr. Allen pushing Mrs. Giles—a sight worthy of pause. He struggled to crawl his own wheelchair forward with his left leg while clinging to her wheelchair with his left hand, he inched them toward the exit. She held her head upright, oblivious to his strife.

I watched him labor through the last twenty feet to the hallway, hail down an employee and signal with all the force of his functioning arm that this lady goes to the hall on the right. He waited to assure they took the correct turn before beginning his own struggle in the opposite direction.

References

PROBLEMS: Vanderbilt University's Sandra Simmons authored studies showing the daily caloric intake of 50 percent to 70 percent of nursing home residents is below recommended levels. She argues, "The issue isn't just food choices but low staffing levels. Many nursing home residents need physical help or, if they have dementia, they need cues or encouragement to eat. If staff members are stretched thin, they might not be able to provide that level of care. And that means that even if there are choices, residents might not get them."

Chapter 13

URINARY INCONTINENCE

Loss of bladder control (urinary incontinence) is a source of fear, shame and depression at any age. For the elderly, incontinence is often the reason for nursing home placement. Caregivers may be unable to manage the difficulties and stress of urinary incontinence at home. Not even confusion and dementia provide escape from the humiliation of lost urinary control; these loved ones often suffer increased anxiety and changes in behavior after such episodes.

The belief that incontinence is an expected consequence of aging is inaccurate. Leaking urine, dribbling and loss of bladder control at any age is not normal. The problem does occur more often in the elderly but it is not an inevitable result of aging. Incontinence is not a disease – it's a symptom. The sooner the disease causing the symptom is diagnosed the greater the chances of successful treatment.

If your loved one enters the nursing home with an incontinence problem, I encourage you to request a diagnosis of the cause. There might be a simple physical explanation. In most instances medical remedies can improve or resolve the loss of control.

If your loved one enters the nursing home without an incontinence problem it is reasonable to expect that they will continue with total urinary control.

Nursing home personnel have a significant impact on every resident's ability to maintain bladder control. Staff responsibilities include hygiene, toileting schedules, toileting assistance, adequate fluids and an individual care plan dedicated to any incontinence problems. Such care requires adequate numbers of nurses and nurse's aides. It is quick and easy for nursing staff to resort to diapers, pull-ups and other commercial products when staffing is short.

The struggle with incontinence often presents a conundrum for residents and their family. Be prepared to become an advocate because your loved one deserves the dignity bladder control affords, and equally, the comfort of appropriate care when urinary control is not possible.

The BE AWARE and BEWARE notes will get you started. An EXAMPLE of persistence follows.

BE AWARE
- Anatomy places women at greater risk for urinary incontinence, but it is no less distressing for men.
- New onset of incontinence in any resident is significant. The cause needs to be identified. Treatment should start when the problem first appears because it becomes more difficult to reverse as time passes.
- Frequent medical problems causing incontinence are urinary tract infections (UTI), constipation and overactive bladder. All are easily treated.
- Bladder and urinary tract infections are a leading cause of incontinence. Sufficient fluids and good genital hygiene are essential for prevention.
- It is reasonable to begin with a simple urinalysis. If infection is present appropriate antibiotics can be ordered. If there is no infection or if antibiotics do not resolve the incontinence then a full urological (urinary) consultation is in order.
- If urology consultation eliminates a medical or physical cause related to the urinary system, staff's responsibility is to develop a care plan aimed at decreasing the resident's incontinent episodes. The care plan will address both physical and mental abilities.
- Physical ailments such as arthritis and strokes may slow down a resident's ability to get to the bathroom. Adequate staffing and patience with these residents supports their efforts to maintain bladder control.
- The cause of incontinent episodes may be long waits for staff assistance. When call lights are not answered promptly a resident's urge to urinate progresses to discomfort, urgency and finally accidents. There is a risk of these residents falling into a pattern of incontinence if they feel efforts to get to the toilet on time are hopeless.
- If incontinence is determined to be the result of declining mental ability, every effort should be made to continue toileting schedules as long as possible. Even occasional success contributes greatly to the resident's self-esteem.

URINARY INCONTINENCE

- Assisting residents to the toilet before and after meals and at bedtime is a simple and effective reminder. Even confused residents usually associate the toilet with urination and empty their bladders thus avoiding the discomfort of a full bladder, urgency and incontinence later.
- A few residents may forget to go to the bathroom, no longer associate the urge to urinate with a toilet or be unable to locate a toilet.
- A resident may be unable to verbalize their need to toilet, but certain mannerisms such as tugging at clothing can identify their need to find a bathroom.
- A personal toileting schedule can sometimes be established. Nursing personnel keep a log of a resident's incontinent episodes for a few days. If there is a recurring pattern of the same incontinent times they can assist them to the toilet prior to the accident.
- Many residents with dementia never experience bladder incontinence when provided appropriate nursing support and medical care.
- Adequate numbers of seasoned staff is the necessary component for prevention of urinary incontinence and encouraging those with intermittent bladder control.
- Residents who are unable to walk or are mostly confined to wheelchairs can still be lifted onto the commode for a toileting schedule.
- A care plan is helpful in limiting foods and drinks which contribute to incontinence: alcohol, chocolate, caffeine, carbonated drinks, sparkling water, chili peppers, artificial sweeteners, spicy foods, sugar or acidic foods, especially citrus fruits. Don't limit water.
- Medications can add to incontinence problems especially heart and blood pressure medicine, sedatives, muscle relaxants and large doses of vitamin C.

BEWARE
- Embarrassment often keeps the elderly from revealing incontinence problems to their personal physician when it first appears. Hence valuable treatment time is lost prior to nursing home admission.

- Sometimes nursing home physicians and nurses simply accept residents' incontinence. They may not be supportive of your request for a urology consultation. However, your loved one's comfort and self-esteem along with your good judgment can guide your decision of whether to insist on a urology consultation, diagnosis and treatment.
- Gerontologists and geriatric urologists are generally more sympathetic and understanding of the elderly's incontinence problems.
- There may be times when recommended surgical procedures or treatments do not warrant risks and hardship for a frail or confused patient.
- Restraints and limited activity are strongly associated with incontinence.
- If transferring a resident to the toilet is impossible, a consistent routine of hygiene, skin care, clothing and linen changes is essential for comfort and prevention of skin breakdown.
- Staff's immediate attention to cleansing and clothing changes after each incontinent incident is necessary to prevent skin rashes, sores and infections; the resident's comfort and self-esteem are equally important.
- Adult diapers and commercial products sometimes become the solution for total incontinence; these products are costly, and the resident most often bears the cost.
- Disposable briefs, pull-ups, etc. come with their own set of limitations; if staff fails to change the resident frequently enough, the same skin problems appear. The resident's skin is at high risk for problems when the disposable product becomes soaked beyond capacity.
- Catheters are not medically acceptable for uncomplicated incontinence. The high incidence of infection and the possibility of trauma place them under scrutiny of state inspectors and federal data collection.

EXAMPLE: How a resident's urinary incontinence caused humiliation and medical professionals' willingness to ignore the problem demanded persistence by a family.

URINARY INCONTINENCE

"Mother you sure look worried." We sat on our usual bench just inside the nursing home entrance. She seemed anxious. Her bottom lip quivered as she mumbled to herself. She leaned forward, looked past me and strained to see outside.

"Mother does your knee hurt?" She could not always communicate her knee pain but answered correctly if asked.

"Oh no, honey. Not bad," she mumbled.

"How about your urine, Mother?" No answer.

Her urinary incontinence was a source of frequent upsets over the past few months. In her previous eighty-eight years, bladder control was never a problem. Nurses' casual responses to my concerns were disheartening. They reasoned, "She's just getting older and her dementia is worse."

One nurse told me, "You should be thankful she's had control this long."

Staff always answered, " We'll get a urine specimen. She could have an infection."

After three normal urine reports I visited with the Director of Nurses. He chided me, "She had you and how many more kids? What do you expect? My wife has five kids and she dribbles every time she climbs stairs. I just tell her, 'Your bladder's paying for all those babies.'"

"Mother, are you still leaking some?" Her bottom lip trembled. She turned away and seemed near tears.

"Mother, when's the last time you had an accident?"

"This morning at the doctor's office. Wet my pants bad."

Doctor's office? Surely not! She is never to go to a doctor's appointment without me. Must be her dementia and confusion.

However, a check with the nurse confirmed a trip to the doctor's office that morning. I asked, "Wanda, isn't there a notation there that I'm to be notified of her doctor's appointments?"

"Well, Frances, you know how it is. They just show up with a list of patients and we're supposed to round them up, get them in the van and over there fast. Nobody had time to call you." I did not doubt Wanda's explanation.

"How long were they over there? Did the doctor say anything about her incontinence? Did he write any new orders?" I asked.

She checked mother's chart. "Well, looks like they were over there a couple of hours. The progress note he sent back says, 'Stable—no changes'. He didn't write any new orders."

"Wanda, it looks to me like they're trying to get Medicare and Medicaid billing out early this month and it's more profitable when they just run them through like cattle, especially if there's a slow day with regular appointments." She nodded her head and smiled. Enough said.

I retreated to ask, "Mother, did you wet your pants before you saw the doctor?"

"I sat on that hard bench an hour before I wet my pants."

"Mother, I am so sorry for all this trouble."

"Don't feel sorry for me. You ought to feel sorry for Jack. Poor old thing's back was hurting so bad he could hardly sit there. Then, he just wet his pants too."

"Mother, were your pants wet when the doctor saw you?"

"My pants, socks and shoes were wet." She twisted her back toward me showing her indignation.

"What did the doctor say?"

"Didn't say nothing. Just slapped that thing over my heart a couple of times. Don't know what he could hear through all my clothes." Mother's clothing was always multilayered and topped off with a fleece jacket zipped to the neck.

"Mother, don't worry. I'll work on this for you."

The next day, I searched for a new doctor. My effort was well rewarded. The new physician, a gerontologist, took an extended history on our first visit, talked with Mother to determine the extent of her dementia and observed her physical ability as Mother slowly but surely followed her instructions to climb onto the examining table. The doctor slipped Mother's shoes and pants off then asked her to raise her knees and spread her legs apart. The doctor's initial look evoked an immediate response. "I can tell you right now why your mother's incontinent. She has a big caruncle."

Without further examination, she patted Mother on the knee and reassured her. "Mrs. Vance you're going to be just fine. We'll get you some medication for this."

Indeed, the first application of her medicated cream resolved Mother's incontinence. There were no more incontinent episodes. During many long road trips, she assumed a sanctimonious attitude and waited in the car during my pit stops. On one occasion she said, "You might need to borrow some of my cream."

References

URINARY INCONTINENCE is estimated to affect 50 to 65 percent of nursing home residents.

URINARY TRACT INFECTIONS (UTI) irritate the bladder wall lining causing strong urges to urinate and sometimes incontinence. The incontinence then increases the risk of repeated urinary tract infections.

CONSTIPATION causes urinary incontinence when hard stool in the rectum irritates shared nerves near the bladder. These nerves become overactive and increase the urge to urinate.

CARUNCLE: small red growth found in the urinary meatus (opening) of females. Other locations are the inner eyelid and underside of the tongue. Differentiate from *carbuncle*, an abscess which may occur anywhere on the body of both men and women.

VOIDING: medical term used often by nursing home staff meaning urination.

CMS Federal Nursing Home Regulations: 483.25(e)(6)(i) The facility must ensure that a resident who is continent of bladder and bowel on admission receives services and assistance to maintain continence unless his or her clinical condition is or becomes such that continence is not possible to maintain.

Medicare.gov/Nursing Home Compare: "Most urinary tract infections can be prevented by keeping the area clean, emptying the bladder regularly, and drinking enough fluid. Nursing home staff should make sure the resident has good hygiene. Finding the cause and getting early treatment of a UTI can prevent the infection from spreading and becoming more serious or causing complications like delirium. It's important to find out whether the UTI is caused by a physical problem, like an enlarged prostate, so proper medical treatment can be given."

HHS Public Access: Gastroenterol Clin North Am. 2008 Sep: Urinary and Fecal Incontinence in Nursing Home Residents. "Urinary and fecal incontinence are co-morbid conditions affecting over 50% of nursing home residents. Both forms of incontinence are risk factors for elderly persons to be placed in the nursing home, and such institutionalization itself is a risk factor for developing incontinence."

US Department of Health and Human Services, Center for Disease Control, June 2014. Prevalence of Incontinence Among Older Adults. https://www.cdc.gov/nchs/data/series/sr_03/sr03_036.pdf

Chapter 14

BOWEL INCONTINENCE

The stresses of caring for a loved one losing bowel control (fecal or stool incontinence) can quickly become overwhelming. Bowel incontinence is not only painful and embarrassing for the individual but also physically and emotionally exhausting for caregivers. We expect to take care of our babies' diapers, but are unprepared to care for parents or a spouse in the same way. The burden of hygiene, soiled clothing, linen changes and laundry are labor intensive, time consuming and expensive. Care becomes more problematic if your loved one is confused, unable to follow instructions or resists care.

A good nursing home's significant benefit is their staff's twenty-four-hour incontinent care. Nurses and nurse's aides are trained to care for incontinence whether a resident suffers an occasional accident or continually leaking stools. Additional responsibility includes nurses checking each resident's bowel habits, developing a plan of care and guiding staff in efforts to decrease bowel problems. Loss of bowel control presents health, emotional and social burdens for both residents and caregivers.

Nursing home admission presents risks of losing regular bowel habits and control because the diet is often lacking in fiber, fewer fluids are accessible and activity decreased. Delayed response to calls for bathroom assistance figures heavily in lost bowel and bladder control. In spite of these barriers residents and their advocates can contribute to staff efforts to prevent and manage incontinence.

Regulatory agencies all agree that residents admitted to a nursing home with bowel incontinence deserve the opportunity to improve control; and those coming to a nursing home with total bowel control merit the dignity of maintaining that control.

The BE AWARE and BEWARE sections offer guidance toward understanding the procedures and routines required to maintain your loved one's bowel control or address problems of incontinence. An EXAMPLE follows.

BE AWARE

- Bowel incontinence is more common in men than women.
- Studies vary in reporting from thirty to fifty percent of nursing home residents experience bowel incontinence. All reports agree that bowel incontinence is associated with increased risk of morbidity.
- There are physical complications caused by incontinent stool's contact with the skin: rashes, itching, burning discomfort, open skin sores progressing to deep, painful wounds and life threatening infections.
- An incontinent stool demands immediate attention and cleansing. The longer the stool is in contact with elderly, delicate skin the greater the probability of skin complications. Enzymes released in the intestines to digest meat are still present in stools and attack skin with the same harshness.
- Emotional consequences of fecal incontinence frequently exceed the physical manifestations. The humiliation of a resident's unpredictable and uncontrolled bowel movement often becomes a barrier to attending activities within the building as well as community visits with family or friends. The solitude of their room is more comfortable than the anxiety and worry of a possible "accident" in public.
- Bladder incontinence usually precedes bowel incontinence but there are many advantages to devoting time and effort toward maintaining bowel control even in the presence of bladder incontinence.
- It is important to inform nurses of your loved one's bowel habits and problems on admission to the nursing home. Bowel status will be a significant factor in the new resident's health and wellbeing.
- Bowel habits occupy a significant place in each resident's care plan with specific strategies for individual problems. However, there is no substitute for a reliable spokesperson. Without advocacy any resident's bowel plan may fall victim to short staffing, employee turnover and lack of supervision. Your loved one's improved self-esteem will greatly reward your efforts.
- I suggest identifying one full-time nurse who shows a willingness to talk to you and answer questions. After he/she realizes you will be consistent in asking questions on each visit or phone call this nurse will take more interest in overseeing the

care plan. Nurse's aides will have invaluable observations of difficulties and successes of an incontinence plan.
- Bowel incontinence demands more than casual acceptance by nursing staff. Nurses' responsibility is to look for causes and develop a care plan with remedies. Their commitment is key to success and any improvement is of great value to a resident.
- Key components of an incontinent care plan and training program focus on individual problems:
    1. What is causing the problem—foods, fluids, medications, inactivity, urgency?
    2. Stool texture—avoid constipation and diarrhea—consider ability to chew, assure adequate fluids, stool softeners, preparations to add bulk?
    3. Toileting schedule?
- Bowel training and retraining programs are dependent on establishing and sticking to a routine over a long period of time.
- Even in the presence of dementia and confusion bowel training programs are worthwhile.
- If a resident's stools are of a normal consistency the solution to incontinence may be as simple as determining what time of day the resident usually has a bowel movement (BM) and arrange a toileting schedule consistent with this time.
- Regular toileting schedules are a mainstay of any incontinence program. Assistance to the restroom on awakening and after meals is a reminder and encourages bowel movements, thus avoiding incontinent episodes. Toileting after warm liquids at breakfast is often successful.
- When diarrhea and frequent stools are associated with incontinence, returning the resident to normal stool consistency is of utmost importance. Diet, medications and bowel diseases may be the culprit. If staff cannot identify and provide solutions a gastrointestinal consultation is in order.
- Constipation is uncomfortable, sometimes painful and a common cause of diarrhea and incontinence; liquid stool leaks around hard, compacted stool in the rectum. Once again the solution is to return to a normal stool consistency. Plenty of fluids, foods with fiber, and stool softeners are preferred solutions.

- Pain medications, muscle relaxants and diuretics (water pills) often cause constipation. Care of residents taking these medications requires daily assessments and an individual plan to avoid severe constipation. Harsh laxatives sometimes used to treat these residents aggravate incontinence.
- Promptness in answering call lights or requests for assistance to the bathroom is essential in preventing incontinent episodes.

BEWARE
- Shaming, threatening or scolding a resident for an incontinent bowel movement is resident abuse and should be handled accordingly.
- The usual dietary principles applied to bowel health are also of utmost importance in the treatment of incontinence. Unfortunately, the nursing home menu may be lacking in fresh fruits and vegetables, beans and whole grains. Poor dental care, missing teeth and ill-fitting dentures may lead a resident to prefer soft foods, puddings and gravy. Staff's persistence varies in assuring adequate amounts of water.
- Bowel incontinence presents significant hurdles for caregivers.
  1. Uncontrolled bowel movements can occur in common areas such as hallways, dining room and treatment areas and can pose the risk of spreading infectious diseases if not cleaned promptly and correctly.
  2. Visitors are very sensitive to odors and soiled clothing, often assuming a negative view of care for even one incident.
- Residents with tube feedings present major problems, usually with diarrhea. Sometimes the best effort is simply to control the consistency of stools especially if the resident is confined to the bed. Feedings with increased fiber content are sometimes helpful. Dieticians may be hesitant to recommend this change if the product is not on the nursing home supplier's contract.
- Residents with dietary supplements and tube feedings are sensitive to changes in commercial brands. Transfers between hospitals and nursing homes may result in a different supply contract, a new feeding brand and increased risk of diarrhea.
- Skin irritations and sores become a major concern when diarrhea is not controlled. Cleaning diarrhea stool from a rectal

rash is painful. Decreasing the number of episodes is a comfort measure for a helpless resident.
- The consultation of a specialized wound care nurse may be needed if skin breakdown develops.

EXAMPLE: This illustration focuses on one daughter's struggle to attain dignity and comfort for her mother through a regular toileting routine. It also shows how toileting programs often fall victim to short staffing.

From my stance in the large circular nurses station I turned to view four long hallways and a shorter entry hall spreading like spokes from a hub at the building's center. The sparkling new building utilized a wagon-wheel floor plan, theoretically allowing greater staff efficiency. One nurse can observe and supervise activity in all hallways simultaneously. Thus staffing a nurse for every one or two halls becomes unnecessary especially during the evening and night shifts.

The rising sun glared through a wall of eastern windows. They framed a lady's silhouette moving briskly toward me. Blinding sunbeams at her back obscured detail beyond a flowing skirt and swinging arms. Physical characteristics became identifiable within a few feet of the nurses station—notably a middle-aged lady with a glare of steel affixed to my eyes. Her determination was evident, as if locking her eyes onto mine assured that I would not walk away while she cleared the distance between us.

As other staff members disappeared, I sensed trouble.

I offered, "Good morning, can I help you?"

"You're new, I haven't seen you before," she answered cautiously.

"Yes, I'm Frances, this is my first day, but I'll be here on weekends. Do you have someone here?"

"I'm Joyce Jacobs, my mother is Anita Anderson in room 432 all the way at the end of the hall. Has anybody told you about my mother?"

"I don't remember anything but I'm trying to learn all the residents. Can I help her with something now?"

"I guess I'm not surprised nobody told you about Mother's problem. I don't think anybody here cares anyway. I brought her here because they told me they'd take her to the bathroom before breakfast. The other place just put diapers on her because they didn't want to bother taking her to the toilet. This place is new, I thought it would be better.

"Mother can't talk and she's confused but I know from taking care of her at home that she'll have a bowel movement if you sit her on the commode before breakfast. She won't have any more stools until you sit her on the commode the next morning. That's how I took care of her bowel incontinence." Her lower lip trembled. She gripped a tissue tightly and paused to regain composure.

"Does she need some help now?" I asked.

She gently shook her head, no. "I really don't think you can help but I want everybody to know how my mother's been treated. I came in at 5:30 Tuesday morning just to see her before work. She'd been left naked on the commode in that cold bathroom, shivering, whimpering and drawn up into a tiny ball with nobody in sight to help. I wrapped her in a robe but could barely get her legs straightened out and walk her back to the wet bed—all this time nobody answered her call light. She's so thin and frail and pitiful and can't ask for help."

Tears cascaded but her penetrating blue eyes remained fixed on me. She was expecting a response. My thoughts raced. *What to say, what to do? Nobody told this daughter they start getting residents dressed for breakfast at 5:00 or 5:30—sometimes earlier if the night shift is short staffed—no answer for the cruelty of leaving a resident alone and naked in the cold—the time needed to strip linen from a wet bed is miniscule—done routinely before leaving the room.*

I began to apologize, "I'm so sorry . . . I'll leave a message for the nursing director . . ."

She interrupted. "I've talked to the nursing director and everybody else. They're a-a-a-a-a-all so sorry and say it won't happen again, but how do I know that? I really don't know unless I come by every morning before work and risk being late—an hour late Tuesday. Anyway, thank you for listening and not making stupid excuses."

She turned sharply and moved swiftly toward the front door. With her exit staff returned to the hub and confirmed the daughter's account as accurate. They added there was only one young, inexperienced nurse's aide working on the hall and she was expected to have twenty-six residents dressed and in the dining room at 7:00 am. The only nurse in the building was busy inside a resident's room at the end of another long hall.

I weighed the chances of success for Mrs. Anderson's bowel program. *Not very good*, I thought. The new building's efficient wagon wheel and promises from management offered little hope without staff. The entire wheel seemed squeaky. Yet, Mrs. Jacob's perseverance with unscheduled visits and clear expectations increase the chances that more of staff's time will be devoted to her mother's bowel program.

References

B&B INCONTINENCE: The combination of lost bowel and bladder control is referred to as B&B incontinence or sometimes, dual incontinence by staff. Bowel movements are referred to as BMs.

RISK: Certain medical conditions such as irritable bowel syndrome, diabetes, dementia, spinal cord injury and neurological disease put residents at higher risk of losing bowel control.

DATA COLLECTION: Regulatory agencies data collection places great emphasis on the prevalence of bowel incontinence within a facility. Inspectors use the following definitions during inspections. https://www.ahcancal.org/facility_operations/Documents/

CONSTIPATION: If the resident has two or fewer bowel movements during the 7-day look-back period or if for most bowel movements their stool is hard and difficult for them to pass (no matter what the frequency of bowel movements). Severe constipation can cause abdominal pain, anorexia, vomiting, bowel incontinence, and delirium. If unaddressed, constipation can lead to fecal impaction.

FECAL IMPACTION: A large mass of dry, hard stool that can develop in the rectum due to chronic constipation. This mass may be so hard that the resident is unable to move it from the rectum. Watery stool from higher in the bowel or irritation from the impaction may move around the mass and leak out, causing soiling, often a sign of a fecal impaction.

Medicare.gov/Nursing Home Compare

U.S. Department of Health and Human Services, Agency for Healthcare Research and Quality, July 2016.
https://effectivehealthcare.ahrq.gov/topics/fecal-incontinence/clinician/

NIH https://www.ncbi.nlm.nih.gov/pubmed/26915601

https://www.ncbi.nlm.nih.gov/pmc/articles/PMC2614622/

https://www.nature.com/articles/ajg2017177
American Journal of Gastroenterology: My approach to Fecal Incontinence: It's all about Consistency (stool, that is) Stacy B. Menees M.D. MS

CHAPTER 15

CONFUSION

When mental changes appear, many terms are used to explain a loved one's need for twenty-four-hour oversight. Descriptions include confusion, dementia and Alzheimer's disease. There may be no clear-cut diagnosis, but simply an inability to manage everyday tasks.

Safety for physically healthy and active individuals often becomes problematic in the presence of wandering, forgetfulness and resistant behaviors. Worry that a meandering loved one will become lost without knowing their own identity, cause a fire by forgetting to turn off stove burners or injure themselves or caregivers during arguments over showers and personal hygiene are only a few of the situations families face daily.

Sorrowful family and friends may question facility placement of a loved one if portions of their mental capacity seem unaffected or mental lapses are intermittent. Health and safety of both the caregiver and the loved one weigh heavily on decisions to seek twenty-four-hour care.

Resident and staff safety determine how each person with mental decline is cared for in a nursing home. Additionally, the nursing home's responsibility is to provide safe care in the least restrictive setting. Many innovative electromagnetic devices such as ankle bracelets, cameras, monitors and special nursing units are available to provide safety and allow freedom of movement.

Perhaps locating appropriate nursing home care for a loved one with mental decline presents the greatest challenge in nursing home selection. Expect the need for oversight to be tedious and long term since many of these residents are quite healthy physically and expected to live a long life.

The BE AWARE and BEWARE sections provide information needed to judge a facility's ability to care for your loved one. Family and staff experiences are captured in the EXAMPLES.

BE AWARE

- Nationally, more than half of all nursing home residents have Alzheimer's disease or another form of dementia.
- Nurse's aides (CNAs) provide eighty to ninety percent of hands-on-care, but they often have minimal job preparation and their training to care for persons with dementia is even more limited.
- Medications are an important component of dementia care and require close oversight and frequent adjustment. Psychiatrists familiar with dementia disorders or gerontologists are usually best at managing medication regimens.
- Consistent nurse staffing is important. Nurses familiar with residents can better evaluate the effects of medications, determine when additional medication or a decrease in medication is needed and communicate observations to family and physician. It is difficult for frequently changing nurses to provide this valuable service.
- Nursing homes utilize technology, innovative programs and building construction to provide care for active residents who no longer have the mental capacity to care for themselves.
- Simple technology includes ankle bands and bracelets that trigger alarms when a wandering resident approaches outside doorways. These devices are not appropriate for residents who can outrun staff.
- Programs promising to limit further mental deterioration warrant close scrutiny. Minimally, you should expect activities and a personalized care plan which allows the resident to utilize their current mental capacity without frustration or anxiety.
- Residents often retain expertise and an interest in their life's work long after they are unable to care for personal needs. Providing a carpenter or mechanic a toy tool box might keep them occupied for hours.
- Specially equipped units within nursing homes currently provide the bulk of care for residents considered a safety risk whether related to wandering or dangerous behaviors.
- Past reference to such areas as the "locked unit" has evolved to the more palatable "secure unit," "special care unit" or simply "the unit." These units have electromagnetically locked doors with keypads, button codes or swipe cards required for opening.

- Trained, regular staff in adequate numbers is of utmost importance for the comfort and stability of the unit's residents. All meals and activities occur within its confines and visitor access is limited. Because the area is isolated from the public's view, secure unit nurses' aides are often sent to other areas of the building when staffing is short. The secure unit is left without adequate staff and impaired residents are unable to report problems.
- Insufficient caregiver numbers result in a great disservice to residents. Anxiety is created by rushed schedules, scarcity of time for personal attention and safety when subtle changes in behavior go unnoticed.
- Regularity in scheduled nurses and nurse's aides prevents resident apprehension caused by the uncertainty of new faces. Regular staff also becomes familiar with resident mannerisms, habits and anxieties, thus they are able to provide early interventions and maintain a calm atmosphere. For example, a resident walking toward his favorite chair now occupied by someone else; regular staff will recognize the potentially volatile situation and invite the sitting resident to come with them for a glass of juice thus clearing the chair for the headstrong resident.
- Organized activities and individual diversion become impossible without adequate numbers of nurse's aides. Units with residents wandering anxiously, rocking aimlessly and staring into space send an undeniable signal of absent care and warehousing.
- Cramped spacing in common areas is not therapeutic. The closeness created by small square footage per resident is a source of agitation for most occupants.

BEWARE
- Nursing home personnel, especially marketing departments, use the terms *Alzheimer's, Special Care Units (SCUs)* and *Memory Care* loosely. You may even hear a simple locked unit referred to as the Alzheimer's unit or SCU. Whether intentionally misleading or staff incompetence, the units referred to often lack the significant upgrades needed to qualify as a licensed or certified Special Care Unit, Alzheimer's, dementia, memory care.

- The Center for Medicare and Medicaid (CMS) provides guidelines for dementia care and encourages their use for state inspections leading to certification and licensure of Special Care Units...inclusive for all dementias. However, only a few states participate in SCU certification programs and hardly any nursing homes can meet the standards: increased staffing numbers and training, resident specific therapies, space, construction, outside activity area and safety features. Therefore, there are few certified or licensed Special Care Units for dementia.
- Certification or licensure of a Special Care Unit for dementia is an addition to the nursing home's regular license to operate. A large number of facilities have designated "units" which lack this certification or licensure. They are unregulated beyond the usual nursing home standards and many are controversial.
- Consumers living in states or areas without certified SCUs are left to compare care based on each facility's self-proclaimed benefits and the recommendations of independent groups. Those caring for elders in any stage of dementia are left to match loved one's needs to individual facility programs.
- Memory care is the trendy term used in current marketing as the industry competes for increasing numbers of aging and their need for dementia care.

EXAMPLES: For these residents expertise in life's work remained intact even after dementia required twenty-four-hour care.

1. I recall one resident, previously the successful owner of a swank restaurant, but no longer able to identify his own personal needs. He offered eloquent reviews of each meal served. Staff learned a great deal about food preparation and presentation by engaging him in mealtime conversation. We memorized his repetitious motto, "presentation is everything" (he relied heavily on parsley, lemon twists, shaved orange peels and cranberries). He would never talk with staff about his profession unless sitting down for a meal.

2. An instance of a military retiree with service as an inspector general stunned staff. He did not know his name, had no idea

where he was and his speech was unintelligible gibberish until he unleashed his opinion of our nurses' station. "A dishonorable boar's nest . . . a wild hog wouldn't claim the mess. If I were inspecting you'd all be relieved of this duty station. But, if you wanted to get ready for my inspection you'd . . . " He railed off a litany of orders.

After we regained our composure his stern authority prevailed. The IG watched, arms folded across his chest as we complied—organizing papers, stacking clipboards, consolidating notes and hiding extra pens and pencils. He tired about the same time staff completed his orders and lapsed back into his previous state of mind.

3. At age fifty-six, Alice seemed far too young for her predicament. For several years we shared registered nurse duties, but she no longer recognized me. Fate placed me as director of nursing at a large nursing home and Alice as a resident in the building's secure unit. She rarely spoke to anyone and even then with only with a few disjointed words. Blank stares met my attempts to talk with her about our work at the V.A. Hospital.

Alice's thinning, auburn hair and petite frame were a familiar sight at the nurses' station. She leaned casually on the surrounding ledge; her penetrating eyes missed nothing. She scrutinized everyone, especially those punching in the security code that opened the locked door. Staff paid her little attention.

The old building's floor plan was unsatisfactory for a secure unit. Two long hallways meandered from a central nurses' station. One ended with a distant lounge shielded from staff view. Residents often gathered there to absorb the afternoon sun beaming through its expansive windows. They enjoyed their view of street traffic and the sidewalk activity only two or three steps away. The exit's keypad lock secured them—they could not open the door and wander into traffic.

On a blistering summer day, a nurse's aide reporting for her afternoon shift paused at my office door. "I think it's great somebody took the unit residents on an outing, but it sure is hot out there."

"Nobody took anybody out!" I replied.

"Well, they're all down at Pampell's corner. Seem to be enjoying it!"

A quick scramble in the van found fifteen residents assembled in a cluster outside the popular antique eatery at the busiest intersection in town. We left Alice in charge of ushering her patients into the van. All were in good condition.

Headcount confirmed and all residents safe, I pieced facts together. Alice learned the exit code by watching employees enter the numbers, or perhaps just listening to conversation. As a registered nurse, she knew the busyness of shift change distracted nurses. She used the opportunity to enter the code and usher the healthy residents onto the city sidewalk. Weak, frail residents were left behind.

Merchants along the several blocks of city street confirmed the group sauntered past their business, did some window shopping, went inside the bank to rest in the plush chairs and air conditioning before moving along.

"The lady in charge ran a tight ship. She made them hold hands and stay together," one observer told me.

With details in hand I faced the task of calling each resident's family and reporting to regulatory agencies. I knew my explanation of Alice's great escape was pretty weak. One last check of the residents found Alice back in her familiar stance at the nurses' station. She seemed proud of her newfound stature among the young nurses.

I said, "Alice, thank you for taking care of the residents today, they needed a good nurse." Her crystal blue eyes locked onto mine. She understood.

EXAMPLE: The heartbreak of a resident's intermittent function and a spouse's emotional conflict.

I noticed a resident's wife blotting her eyes as she left the secure unit. As usual, Mrs. Alexander was visiting during her lunch hour. Her sophisticated business suit and confident stride belied her inner turmoil. As I approached she stopped to talk with me.

"You won't believe what he just said to me," she wept while trying to salvage her mascara. "He just said, 'I love you' and that's the first thing he's said to me in months."

"I know he recognizes you. He looks straight at you and tries to talk," I said.

"I feel so bad because I can't take him home but I have to work and pay these bills."

"You're doing the right thing, keep coming every day and visit any time—day or night. If you're uneasy call the unit and check on him."

"I know. It's just so hard." She assured me with a raised hand and step toward the door. It seemed more like a stride to preserve her emotions than a return to work.

EXAMPLE: The value of regular staff, familiar to residents, is evident in this situation.

Jake did not like to shower. He preferred to pace along the unit's baseboard perimeter…the same path the exterminator took for monthly service calls. Jake was adamant. When approached for a shower the headstrong pacing began. Episodes of behavioral outbursts and fighting persisted until Julie decided to pace with him. She devised a method of stacking clean clothes, towel and washcloth in a neat bundle, held close to her chest on their path around the unit. A few feet before the shower room door Julie extended the bundle in front of Jake, but was careful not to touch him or interrupt his stride. He understood the routine and Julie allowed him to continue his path, with her alongside, until he finally accepted the bundle and careened into the shower room, never breaking stride. He showered and dressed himself with Julie on standby.

Sometimes Julie made three or four silent passes with Jake before he accepted her bundle. He would not accept the bundle from anyone else. On Julie's days off we determined Jake did not need a shower.

References

KAISER FAMILY FOUNDATION: According to their 2013 report, Implementation of Affordable Care Act Provisions to Improve Nursing Home Transparency, Care Quality, and Abuse Prevention, "Direct care workers with little or no training in dementia care may misinterpret residents' behavior as aggression, rather than as symptoms of their disease or inability to communicate their needs. Heavy workloads may also increase nursing assistants' stress levels and further inhibit their ability to interpret and address behavioral symptoms that are caused by residents' disease or inability to communicate pain, fear, and other needs."

THE AFFORDABLE CARE ACT: The ACA requires nurse's aides to be trained in dementia care within their 75 hours of basic CNA training. CMS provides each Medicare and Medicaid nursing home a six-hour curriculum for initial and in-service training. The high turnover of nursing assistants creates a continuing challenge to maintain a trained direct care workforce.

ALZHEIMER'S ORGANIZATION: Dementia Care Practice Recommendations for Assisted Living Residences and Nursing Homes:
https://www.alz.org/national/documents/brochure_DCPRphases1n2.pdf

JOINT COMMISSION: The Joint Commission is an independent group administering voluntary accreditation programs for health care organizations. Their *accreditation* programs are not associated with Medicare and Medicaid *certifications* or state inspection *licensures*. In 2014 Joint Commission introduced their accreditation program for memory care in Nursing Care Centers (assisted living and nursing homes) and certification credentials for individual staff members. The organization's emphasis is on quality indicators. Although the group is non-profit, the accreditation process is quite expensive for nursing homes applying for the accreditation. The facility must bear the cost of Joint Commission programs including manuals, training materials, and on-site inspections.
    http://www.jointcommission.org/assets/1/6/R3_MemoryCare_Accreditation_Requirements.pdf

CHAPTER 16

RESTRAINTS

The mention of restraint use in nursing homes stirs strong opinions focused on abuse, safety and ethics. Emotions enter the picture when your loved one is the center of a restraint discussion. Sometimes you may feel a restraining device (vest, lap belt, etc.) is needed to protect from falls when nurses say no restraint should be used. At other times restraint use may seem to be a convenient substitute for inadequate staffing.

Anything restricting a resident's free movement is considered a restraint. Nursing home regulations and practices categorize restraints as either physical or chemical. Both may be in use on the same resident.

A few physical restraints are obvious: belts, vests and wrist straps anchoring the resident to a chair or bed, padded mittens, lap belts, backward tilted recliners, bars through wheelchair spokes and brakes preventing movement, trays placed over chairs to obstruct standing, bedrails, tightly tucked sheets, being locked in a room, electronic surveillance and alarms.

Chemical restraints - medications - are less obvious. In general, drugs used to treat depression, psychosis and anxiety, stabilize moods, induce sleep or a calming effect, fall into the category of chemical restraints.

Today, state laws and federal regulations limit the use of restraints to the treatment of medical conditions. In addition to the resident's medical need, a series of decisions is associated with the use of any restraint whether physical or chemical - a physician's order along with a medical explanation for the order, an Informed Consent signed by the resident's responsible party and a comprehensive care plan.

Limiting a resident's free movement requires thoughtful consideration of risks and benefits. Dangers of restraint use include injury and accidental death. On the other hand, medications considered chemical restraints allow many residents to function well and enjoy life within the nursing home. Your loved one is unique.

Many individual factors will enter your decision to support or reject restraint use.

The following BE AWARE and BEWARE sections provide further insight as you make that decision. An EXAMPLE follows.

BE AWARE
- The National Institute of Health reports the use of physical restraint use in nursing homes varies from 4 to 85 percent.
- The number of restraints in use is usually related to staffing numbers. The fewer direct care staff the more restraints will be used.
- Physical restraints have sometimes been described as positioning, safety and protective devices, also reminders for impulsive residents. The terms may seem more palatable, but they remain restraints.
- Velcro fastening devices have been promoted as easy-release, therefore not really a restraint. However, dementia or helplessness may block a resident's ability to loosen them. They are restraints.
- Alarms attached to beds, chairs or clothing are among the least restrictive of restraints; they sound when the resident attempts to stand. Adequate staff and quick responses to alarms are essential for their success. Wily residents think nothing of leaving them screeching as they make their way to the bathroom.
- Any device used to interfere with a resident's feeling, fiddling, scratching or tugging at bandages or tubes (catheters, tubing delivering oxygen, nutrition, intravenous fluids and medications) is a restraint.
- Forcibly holding or limiting a resident's movement for a medical examination, treatment, shower, dressing or grooming is also a restraint.
- There are risks associated with restraint use: falls, incontinence, constipation, bruises, skin tears, pressure sores, joint stiffness, decreasing ability to walk and use muscles, reduced bone mass, depression, agitation, lost dignity, strangulation from straps and bedrails, discomfort and pain.
- Federal and state regulations require physical restraints to be checked for problems every hour and released for ten minutes

every two hours. The resident must be repositioned by staff and given a chance to move and go to the toilet.
- Use of physical restraints, even for medical reasons, requires close attention to a resident's comfort, safety, need for fluids, toileting, exercise and social interaction.
- Drugs become chemical restraints when they are not used for medical purposes. Providing a resident safety and comfort is a medical use. Safety includes the ability to concentrate and co-operate with a treatment plan. Residents become more comfortable when anxiety and fears are relieved.
- Medications become chemical restraints when used for staff convenience or discipline. An example would be sedating a resident for unruly behavior or resistance when therapy, activities and a targeted care plan are needed. Lack of manpower may influence decisions to use chemical restraints instead.
- Each nursing home resident has a right to be free from unnecessary medication (chemical restraint) defined as: excessive dosage, excessive lengths of time, without a medical purpose, without adequate monitoring or considering serious side effects.
- Facilities have a right to determine whether they care for a resident who rejects medications for behaviors dangerous to other residents or staff.
- Restorative nursing care is recognized as an effective alternative to restraints. In these programs, the restorative nurse's aide's time is devoted to maintaining or improving residents' functional level. Guided by a registered nurse or licensed therapist, they help residents with exercise plans: walking, balance, safe transfers from beds and wheelchairs, muscle strengthening and range of motion, walker safety, bowel and bladder training programs and self-help activities. This care promotes safety, strength and self-reliance. Each facility has a restorative program but few assign more than minimal hours for a restorative nurse's aide.

BEWARE
- Restraints are a leading cause of incontinence.

- Fall prevention is the most often used reason for restraints. Research demonstrates that restraints do not prevent falls. If a restrained resident falls they are more likely to be seriously injured than if they fell without restraints. Examples: turning a wheelchair over while restrained in it, strangulation from ties and straps.
- Full-length bedrails are among the most dangerous of restraints; Entrapment, strangulation, hanging and fall injuries occur when residents try to get out of bed. A safer solution is lowering the bed and placing padding on the floor for a resident prone to rolling out of bed. Newer bed designs with half-rails extending from head to waist when raised are a good solution. Residents can grab the rails to turn over or easily sit on the bedside with feet solidly on the floor.
- There are dangers associated with the use of any restraint, physical or chemical. Before an Informed Consent is signed, the nursing home's responsibility is to *inform* the responsible party of the risks associated with the use of each restraint.
- Informed Consent forms are also legal cover for the nursing home.
- Federal and state guidelines for restraint use are strict and inspector's guidelines for enforcement are stringent. Electronic data collection generates the percentage of restraints in use for each facility. Of more importance to the nursing home is the emphasis placed on decreasing percentages. A nursing home may never get to zero percentage, but trials of decreased usage (decreasing times residents spend restrained whether physical or chemical) improves facility percentages. Statistics often become more important than a resident's wellbeing in efforts to improve these percentages.
- Regulatory agencies collect data on each facility's use of medications with potential to become chemical restraints. Monthly pharmacist reviews focus on these medications. Most facilities attempt to show good faith by reducing dosages and the overall number of residents receiving medications for depression, psychosis, anxiety, mood swings and sleep even when they are used for medical conditions.
- Resident-on-resident violence has increased in recent years. One resident's right to be free from physical or chemical

restraints is not more important than the safety of other residents or staff. So far, the nursing home industry has not provided staffing numbers and training needed for early detection and injury prevention. The result is that facilities lean toward one resident's right to be free from restraints over another's right to safety. When violent behavior has resulted in death of another resident their legal defense is that the facility was just following the law. Responsibility is deflected to the violent resident and law enforcement as a homicide.

- Some facilities advertise as "restraint-free." A restraint-free facility requires increased staffing ratios with additional training and selective admissions. Too often nursing homes use "restraint-free" as a marketing tool without committing additional resources. If your loved one is injured in a restraint-free nursing home the defense in legal actions will be that the injured resident or responsible party knew the facility did not restrict residents' freedom. Therefore, liability rests with the injured resident.
- During my career of extensive travel and consultations across the spectrum of nursing home organizations, I'm aware of only one facility fulfilling the commitment to a safe, restraint-free environment.

EXAMPLE: This illustration could be used in several chapters, but is placed here to show an instance of *medical symptoms* and need for physical restraints. The situation also shows the pitfalls of not visiting a facility in advance and depending upon hospital staff for transfer arrangements.

I was thankful for the long hallway. I moved at a snail's pace from our new resident's room toward the nurse's station. I needed time to formulate a response for his wife; she leaned on the ledge surrounding the desk, awaiting answers. *How could this happen?*

I pieced the situation together with information from the ambulance attendants, the unit's charge nurse, the new resident, and his son. Mr. Logan arrived on the ambulance stretcher with a vest restraint in place because his medical condition required that he lie almost flat in bed. He could have his head rolled up slightly, but only in bed. He could not be allowed to sit on the side of the bed nor stand up. When he attempted to do so, he passed out, seizures began and progressed to severe, prolonged episodes. The seizure attacks are described as life threatening because the symptoms always progressed to breathing problems.

Mrs. Logan told staff, "He's fast when he needs to get up and he needs a restraint for his safety and protection." The nurse called me for help because our facility had a restraint-free policy.

I found Mr. Logan to be anxious, made worse by the unfamiliar surroundings and strangers. He was disheveled, curly black hair hung over his ears and neck in ringlets. He looked as though he hadn't slept for days. Attempted conversation netted only a few unintelligible words and increased anxiety. He waved his hands, gestured and smiled inappropriately.

The hospital's transfer report identified a fall risk and called for a low bed, so his bed frame rested only a few inches off the floor. The ambulance attendants retrieved their vest restraint. His young son, a strapping 6'4", moved a chair to his father's bedside, rested his chin in his hands, braced his elbows on his knees and peered down at his father. He became the protector while his father babbled nonsensically. Dad would not be getting out of bed on his watch.

Our nursing home's restraint (physical) free policy allowed only self-release belts. Theoretically, the resident is not restrained because he/she can undo the attached Velcro or snap-on belt at any time. A belt around Mr. Logan's waist would not prevent him from sitting up in bed and his dementia stood in the way of his understanding the device or remembering any instructions to lie flat. The facility policy did not allow for medically necessary restraints.

The calmness exuded by Mrs. Logan's blue pantsuit and tasteful accessories from a distance was betrayed by the up close physical, mental and emotional stress portrayed on her face. My conversation with Mrs. Logan revealed an insightful caregiver, knowledgeable of his condition and articulate in stating his needs. She was not angry with staff, or anyone for that matter, "I'm just trying to get help for my husband. He's been in the hospital for two weeks."

Because the medical need was obvious, I thought there might be an exception for Mr. Logan. My Sunday call to the Director of Nursing only supported the facility's policy. The family had no one who could sit with him twenty-four hours a day…the condition for him staying in the nursing home. Mrs. Logan understood we must send him back to the hospital.

At this point I could only guess at what happened and apologize to Mrs. Logan. The hospital was probably rushing to discharge their patient after a two-week admission. The nursing home failed to obtain all the information needed before accepting a resident. Now locating a nursing home for her husband would start all over again. I encouraged her to visit the next facility and use her own good judgment about the best place for her husband.

References

REGULATIONS: CMS Federal Nursing Home Regulations: 483.13(1) Restraints. The facility must ensure that the resident is free from physical or chemical restraints imposed for purposes of discipline or convenience and that are not required to treat the resident's medical symptoms. When the use of restraints is indicated, the facility must use the least restrictive alternative for the least amount of time and document ongoing re-evaluation of the need for restraints.

Additional Federal guidelines:
"Physical Restraints" are defined as any manual method or physical or mechanical device, material, or equipment attached or adjacent to the resident's body that the individual cannot remove easily and which restrict freedom of movement or normal access to one's body. "Convenience" is defined as any action taken by the facility to control a resident's behavior or manage a resident's behavior with a lesser amount of effort by the facility and not in the resident's best interest.
"Medical Symptom" is defined as an indication or characteristic of a physical or psychological condition.

CMS will hold the facility accountable for the appropriateness of that determination. The physician's order alone is not sufficient to warrant the use of the restraint. It is further expected, for those residents whose care plans indicate the need for restraints, that the facility engage in a systemic and gradual process toward reducing restraints (e.g., gradually increasing the time for ambulation and muscle strengthening activities).

National Institute of Health.

https://www.ncbi.nlm.nih.gov/pmc/articles/PMC2564468/

http://www.nursinghomeabuseguide.org/neglect/chemical-restraints

https://www.agingcare.com/questions/protect

Providermagazine.com

Provider Magazine: VOL. 42, No. 2, February 2016, "Resident-on-Resident Violence Draws Attention."

CHAPTER 17

CARE PLANS

Each nursing home resident has a recorded care plan. This document identifies that resident's individual problems whether physical, mental or social. Some of these problems will be the reason for nursing home admission; others may be simple resident preferences such as food choices. Example problems you might find on care plans are poor appetite, incontinence, generalized weakness, cannot speak, wanders at night, anxiety, pain and many others. The list of problems is a collaboration of the resident, staff and responsible party observations. The difficulties identified are specific and personal for each resident.

Once problems are identified, the collaborative effort begins a plan to care for each problem, thus the term *care plan*. The resident care plan is a professional road map quite similar to an architect's blueprint or a teacher's lesson plan. It maps a step-by-step guide to staff's approach and the care they provide for each problem.

Finally, the care plan team establishes a goal for each problem whether the expectation is to resolve, improve, or just maintain the present status.

The care plan begins on admission with physician's orders and nurse's observations entering into a basic plan within forty-eight hours. Everyone involved in the resident's care (social service, dietary, nursing, activities and therapy) adds observations in the following days, then staff meets to discuss and finalize a plan of care. The resident and the responsible party are invited to the meeting; their observations are very important.

It is helpful to understand that care plan meetings do not focus on medical diagnosis but the problems caused by a diagnosis or sometimes just general concerns. Even though a physician is managing medical care, the staff will need to plan care for the symptoms experienced by the resident. Examples: a heart attack diagnosis but the nursing home problem is a resident too weak to walk, a stroke patient no longer able to talk, an arthritis diagnosis with the resident experiencing joint pain, or a diabetes diagnosis needing a special diet and skin care. For non-medical problems no one is better prepared to offer observations than the resident and family—sleep habits, food dislikes, toileting schedules.

The care plan is a basic tool used by regulatory agencies to evaluate resident care during routine inspections and complaint investigations. The significance of care plans is underscored by professional responsibilities and licenses - nurses, therapists, social workers, dieticians and the nursing home's license to operate. The complexity and frequency of care identified in the care plan influences Medicare and Medicaid payments. As a legal nursing consultant, I found care plans to be among nursing homes' greatest vulnerabilities.

Care plans are explained further in the BE AWARE and BEWARE sections. EXAMPLES follow.

BE AWARE
- Care plans are discussed, created and finalized at scheduled meetings.
    1. Participants include a representative from every department involved in the resident's health care: nursing, therapy, dietary, activities, social service, nursing assistants, the resident and responsible party.
    2. The social worker is usually in charge of family contacts and meeting schedules.
    3. Care plan meetings are scheduled within twenty-one days of admission and every ninety days thereafter. Interim meetings may be called if problems arise.
    4. Although scheduled during regular business hours, the nursing home staff has some obligation to accommodate the responsible party's availability.
    5. Care plan meetings may be held in the resident's room if they are alert but cannot be transported to a meeting room.
    6. Care plan meetings identify specific health care issues, decide if staff intervention is needed and map a course for such intervention. The same problems may have different goals and approaches for each individual.
    An example:
        Problem: Very weak—needs help to stand

CARE PLANS

Goal: Decrease weakness—stand alone

Plan:
1. Get a dietary consult to check nutritional status.
2. Provide extra fluids at mealtime and in. supplemental treats.
3. Assist with all transfers out of bed and walking.
4. Begin a fall risk program to prevent injury.
5. Get physical therapy consult to establish an exercise schedule.
6. Encourage participation in activities.

Another example of the same problem:
Problem: Very weak—needs help to stand
Goal: Comfort and safety
Plan:
1. Get a dietary consult to determine food preferences.
2. Offer extra fluids and between meal treats.
3. Provide assistance with transfers out of bed, toileting and bathing.
4. Begin a fall risk program to prevent injury.

- The individual care plan is always evolving.
  1. Multiple problems are listed for each resident.
  2. During care plan meetings each problem is reviewed.
  3. Participants decide whether the plan for each problem is working, needs adaptations or is resolved with the goal attained.
  4. New problems are entered as the process continues.
- Staff time for care plan meetings is limited.
  1. Each staff member reviews resident records and prepares their own contribution before the meeting.
  2. In many instances staff enters a resident problem into a computer program to generate a textbook care plan designed to address any question raised by an inspector. Additional nursing home benefit of such programs is saved staff time and thought. Recent rule changes stress a more personalized approach.
  3. Be prepared to pinpoint your own concerns, solutions and requests.

4. Do not expect much discussion. Instead staff will probably give you their observations and solutions and hope you agree.
  5. It is your right to object to any plans presented by staff.
- The focus of care plan meetings is health care; they are not the place for complaints about housekeeping, laundry, the menu, a bill or any other operational issue.
- Nursing homes are required to notify the responsible party of scheduled care plan meetings, but rarely emphasize the need for their participation. Sometimes notifications arrive late. A call to the social worker or activities director may be needed if the ninety-day review is approaching and a notice has not arrived.
- If you are unable to attend meetings, be sure to relay problems to the social worker and follow with a written note or communication supporting your conversation.
- When a responsible party does not attend care plan meetings or communicate with its professionals they miss an opportunity to promote a loved one's interests. Expect this absence to become an issue when problems arise. The facility's defense: "Nobody told us" or "They ignored care plan notices."

BEWARE
- Routine inspections, complaint investigations and reimbursement audits assure staff attention to care plans.
- A resident problem without a care plan does not bode well with inspectors.
- Problems recorded in care plans but ignored by staff are a major infraction during inspections and complaint investigations.
- If a resident is harmed or their condition deteriorates because of either situation above, the nursing home can face a major inquiry by regulatory agencies.
- A few nursing homes conduct care plan meetings as intended with utmost interest in the best resident care. A majority considers the care plan an exercise of paper compliance. You will be able to tell the difference.
- Nursing homes embrace the efficiency of computer generated care plans: enter a problem, constipation for example, and a textbook care plan is produced within seconds. These care plan

designs are detailed and far too comprehensive for facilities to achieve.
- Short staffing often leaves employees unable to provide the care specified in the care plan's design and accurate documentation becomes almost impossible. In an oversimplification: a resident with a care plan problem of constipation dies from a bowel obstruction; the nursing home's responsibility is detailed in the care plan; the care was not followed as evidenced by their own faulty or absent documentation, therefore adding weight to a claim that failure to follow the care plan contributed to the resident's death.
- Documentation pages generated to match the care plan are designed to assure that staff verifies each detail of care was completed during their shift. Many are computerized, allowing employees to quickly click through the list. Considered to be fail-safe documentation systems they do not take into consideration the inaccuracies of poorly trained staff, turnover, attempts to teach new staff and short staffing. In too many instances patient care time is sacrificed for documentation; more time is spent recording the care than is used to provide the care. Far too often residents do not receive documented care.
- 2016 rules issued by The Center for Medicare and Medicaid (CMS) requires more person-centered care plans focusing on personal and cultural diversity. The new regulations place emphasis on each resident's involvement and control of their own care plan. Additional training and staffing are necessary to fulfill care plans based on individual resident preferences. The rules began phasing into practice in 2017. Nursing home industry spokespersons have resisted the new rules citing the cost of training and the increased number of caregivers needed. (As we go to print, CMS has delayed implementation of the rule changes until 2019.)

EXAMPLE: An administrator's way of dealing with the necessity of care plans which he seemed to consider paper compliance rather than an interest in resident care.

Many nursing home workdays start in the administrator's office with a stand-up gathering of all facility department heads, nursing, laundry, housekeeping, activities, dietary, maintenance and sometimes the receptionist. Stand-up because there are not enough chairs to seat everyone and the comfort of a seat might tempt someone to prolong the meeting. Typically, the administrator questions each department head about their schedule for the day and what they plan to accomplish by day's end.

I recall attending one such meeting while filling in during the regular Director of Nursing's vacation. As the administrator wound down the meeting he asked, "Okay, this is care plan day, how many do we have?"

"Six," answered the activities director.

"How many families are coming," he questioned.

"Three families," she responded.

"Can you get the families out in fifteen minutes?" the administrator's eyes moved around the room directing contact at each care plan member.

"Sure, of course," staff answered in unison.

"Agnes," the administrator said to the receptionist, "Don't forget to watch the clock. Knock on the door if they're not out in fifteen minutes—just tell them another family's waiting."

"Yes sir. I understand."

"Now I figure care plans should be done in one and a half hours so everyone can get back on their jobs. Agreed?"

There were no dissents, the care plan meeting room stood empty within the allotted time.

Regrettably, the idea that time spent talking with families and devising a workable care plan is a waste of staff time dominates in the industry. Computer generated care plans are meant to be a foolproof mechanism for regulatory inspections. In many instances computer care plans are so detailed and complex it is impossible for staff to provide such extensive care. The result is more inspection problems and potential litigation because technology has recorded a plan that staff cannot fulfill. Recent regulation changes dictate more individualized care plans with personal care staff (nurse's aides) participation and resident preferences.

EXAMPLE: This situation characterizes the intent of care plans and the importance of family participation.

During her long residency in a small South Texas nursing home, Viola projected a delightful spirit to her caregivers and peers. An ideal resident until hospitalized for pneumonia, she returned to the nursing home in a weakened state. Attentive staff realized she could eat very little, sipped only small amounts of liquids and rarely talked. Viola's normally thin body seemed unable to survive even a few pounds of weight loss.

Lab work ordered by her physician revealed severe malnutrition. Critical decisions needed to be made in view of Viola's limited ability to understand and communicate. The social worker arranged a care plan meeting with her nephew, the responsible party. He lived a distance away, rarely visited and seemed unfamiliar to staff.

The young man, early twenties, arrived the next day and visited Viola before the meeting. He listened intently as staff reviewed her problems and offered choices for care: (1) no intervention and hope she gets better, (2) call hospice if she does not start eating in a few days or (3) insert a feeding tube.

His response, "I know about feeding tubes, the good and all the philosophical objections. I think my auntie deserves a chance to get better. I'm a farmer . . . I don't let my livestock starve and I don't want my Auntie to be hungry."

The social worker tried delicate confirmation, "Then you want a feeding tube for Viola?"

"Yes. Absolutely, but I don't want one of those things stuck down her nose, I want a good, soft tube punched straight into her stomach."

The remainder of the meeting moved as rapidly as the beginning. A plan was quickly devised to schedule for tube placement, have a registered dietician recommend tube feedings to correct her malnutrition, gradually decrease the amount of tube feedings as she became strong enough to eat, and remove the feeding tube when she was eating adequately. Additionally, staff recommended a psychiatric consultation for possible depression . . . he readily agreed.

Within two days she was receiving an antidepressant and feedings via a stomach tube . . . no attached bags, tubing, machines or wires . . . just one soft tube tucked comfortably beneath clothing and exposed only when nurses provided her nutritional supplement.

Viola's next ninety-day care plan review documented her eating full meals in the dining room, enjoying her friends and participating in activities again. Her psychiatrist recommended continuing her antidepressant and her feeding tube was scheduled for removal.

The care plan for the next ninety days focused on assuring adequate nutrition.

EXAMPLE: This care plan meeting shows how facility staff may associate a resident's need with payment sources. In this case staff did not see a benefit in equipment they associated with facility responsibility, but it became a good idea when the family assumed responsibility for purchase.

A well-prepared staff gathered for Mother's quarterly care plan meeting. The nurse, activities director, food service manager, social worker and physical therapist each reviewed their portion of chart data: age, stable weight, forgetfulness, knee discomfort, uses walker, confusion. Based on their observations most of the care plan should be continued for another ninety days with only a question and a problem.

The social worker questioned Mother's resuscitation status. "We still have Mrs. Vance as a full code—meaning you wish her to have full resuscitative measures if we find her not breathing."

"Yes, vigorous resuscitation, EMS and transport to the hospital," I replied.

"Well, you know she's getting more confused so we always consider quality of life in a person with dementia," he challenged.

"So far, Mother seems happily confused and her family and medical power of attorney are in total agreement—she needs to be resuscitated." Although tired of this habitual question I expected it to surface again.

The nurse chimed in, "Actually, there's a safety issue with Mrs. Vance. She won't wear her slippers when she gets up at night—she's a real fall risk especially since she wears her socks to bed. Sometimes she wanders into the hall looking for a nurse. The slick floors and slick socks are a bad combination."

I asked, "What do you think we should do? She knows her no-skid slippers are beside the bed." *I thought, this is not a new problem, it comes up at every care plan meeting.*

"Sometimes she forgets to put her shoes on during the day," noted the activities director.

"Will she put shoes on if you remind her?" I asked.

"Yes, during the day she will thank us for the reminder and put shoes on. But she told the night nurse, 'Never did wear shoes to the bathroom at night and I ain't startin' now.' She wants to keep the socks on . . . said her feet are cold. She's also had some choice comments about the air conditioning." The observations brought chuckles from the group.

"Maybe I can find some bulky, non-skid socks for her to wear at night. She likes wild socks so maybe if they're wild enough she'll try them," I proposed. The group agreed and continued the plan of gentle reminders when found without her shoes or slippers.

As they readied to wind down the meeting someone asked if I had any questions. "Yes, I was wondering if one of the new rolling walkers would be helpful to Mother? You know, the small, black ones with a seat. I thought Donna (physical therapist) might be able to tell me if Mother could manage one safely."

Donna replied, "Well, the nursing home does not provide the new walkers only the simple, standard ones."

"I know, but I'm just not sure she can manage one. Would it just make her more confused?" Again, I directed my question to Donna. *After all, I thought, this is her area of expertise.*

"Medicare and Medicaid don't pay for medical equipment for nursing home residents." Donna seemed defensive.

I thought, an humble, "please-help-me" approach might work. "Well, I guess I just need help figuring out if the new walker would work for Mother. I know they come in different sizes and models but I don't know much about walkers. I'm sure Donna knows better. I don't expect anybody to pay for it. Just thought I'd go buy it if it will help her."

"Oh, yes! I think she would really enjoy it. No safety issues and she can sit down more often taking some pressure off her knee." Financial questions relieved, Donna now seemed enthusiastic.

"Great, I'll work on it," I replied. The recommendation for a new walker entered into Mother's care plan.

Noteworthy components of this meeting hold true for most care plan meetings. Nursing homes prefer Do Not Resuscitate orders, feeling that it simplifies their job. There is always an effort to shift any safety issue (socks/fall) to a resident or family responsibility thus freeing the nursing home of blame if an injury occurs. Most nursing homes feel no obligation to provide special equipment and may go to extraordinary lengths in support of their position such as denying a need or blaming Medicare and Medicaid for not paying for equipment. In fact, medical equipment has been figured into the daily room rate paid by Medicare and Medicaid.

References

PROPOSED REFORM NOW DELAYED TO 2019: CMS3260-P Reform of Requirements for Long-Term Care Facilities On day 1, facility staff also begins to assess the resident and to identify problems. Both activities provide the core process, as staff look at issues of safety, nourishment, medications, ADL needs, continence, psychosocial status and so forth. Facility staff determines whether or not there are problems that require immediate intervention (e.g., providing supplemental nourishment to reverse weight loss or attending to a resident's sense of loss at entering the nursing facility). For each problem, facility staff will focus on causal factors and implement an initial plan of care based on their understanding of factors affecting the resident.

CHAPTER 18

THEFT

Theft of resident's possessions varies from an ever-present problem in some nursing homes to a rare occurrence in a handful of facilities. It is difficult to isolate thieves. Around-the-clock activity of routine care mixed with the circulation of staff, visitors and residents, exposes belongings to many individuals thus creating multiple suspects.

A greater possibility is that items are simply misplaced during the hustle and bustle of nursing home operations. Whether disappearing during laundry and cleaning cycles, misplaced during routine care or stolen, each incident creates resident turmoil.

Personal articles brought to the nursing home are treasured reminders of their life's journey and often the resident's only remaining possessions. The unsettling loss of these belongings can result in troublesome health symptoms: stress, anxiety, depression and blood pressure changes to name a few.

Daily routines put staff in contact with a resident's belongings whether nursing, laundry, housekeeping, maintenance or social service. Employees can betray this access with theft. Families usually understand how their loved ones' articles become lost during routine care but are at a loss when stealing becomes evident, especially small items of little monetary value.

Nursing home ownership and the administrator determine each facility's response to theft complaints—sometimes sympathy and always denial of a thief among employees. Unless a resident's representative persistently seeks answers theft is ignored. The end result will always be a total denial of any nursing home responsibility.

The BE AWARE and BEWARE sections provide insight into theft within nursing homes and a few suggestions for prevention. EXAMPLES follow.

BE AWARE
- Among the stack of papers signed on admission is a *Release of Responsibility* for personal possessions. The document states that

the facility is not responsible for any article brought into the building. The purpose is to shift total financial and legal accountability for disappearance or damage to the resident.
- An inventory of personal items is compiled on admission. The list is helpful in identifying things misplaced between residents and proof of ownership in cases of theft. Although rarely maintained over a long period of time, the inventory is helpful in verifying ownership of distinctive items such as watches. The nursing home still relies on the Release of Responsibility document to avoid any obligation for items on the list.
- A nursing home's first response to theft complaints is predictable. Administrators attempt to divert attention from probable theft to other possibilities: an unknown, wandering resident picked up the article and put it somewhere else; the forgetful owner misplaced it; the article will show up in the laundry; it was accidentally tossed into the trash or visitor theft. Any hint of a thief among staff will be dismissed along with denying other thefts in the building.
- Administrators may suspect or know the identity of a thieving employee while denying the thefts. They usually terminate the staff member for trivial reasons thus avoiding the messiness of legal action by the guilty (proving the charge), reports to licensing agencies and law enforcement.
- Ignoring thefts keeps the nursing home out of local police reports and newspapers. There is no mention on the suspect's employment record allowing them to move on to another facility.
- Fellow staff members are also victims of theft. They often suspect or know the culprit's identity. It is upsetting to have cash or valuables stolen from their purses and bags when they feel that their employer knows the thief's identity.
- Frequent changes in employment hinder identification of offenders. When the guilty employee feels suspect they move on to another facility.
- Jewelry is especially susceptible to loss and theft because of its value and size—too small to be labeled with a name and easily concealed during theft. Wearing jewelry is not a safeguard as many believe.

1. Watches, bracelets and necklaces are usually removed during showers and in danger of being forgotten on a shower room shelf, then disappearing or becoming lost in a linen barrel.
2. Consider costume substitutes for a jewelry lover and bring originals for special occasions only.
3. Unconsciousness presents an opportunity to remove rings held in place for many years by knotty, twisted knuckles. Rings disappearing between the time a resident becomes comatose and the arrival of an ambulance or death and the mortician's arrival are especially heartbreaking.

- Designer clothing and accessories are best brought to the nursing home for special events and returned home afterward.
- A facility-wide search is sometimes initiated if a resident's family persists in seeking answers or if many articles throughout the building seem misplaced. Findings usually include lost clothing, dentures and eyeglasses in the wrong resident's room but rarely items reported as thefts.
- Staff knows which confused residents tend to pick up and carry articles from room to room and observe for the behavior. Conscientious employees also become familiar with each resident's possessions and return them to the owner if found in the wrong room. Marking each resident's belongings is helpful.
- Residents do not give up their right to police protection upon entering a nursing home. A theft report to local law enforcement is an option if nursing home administration ignores complaints.

BEWARE
- There is no way to determine the prevalence of theft within a facility. If administration denies employee theft or any responsibility they feel no need to keep track of complaints. Records run the risk of providing a trail for possible investigation or litigation.
- Anything left with a nursing home resident is an open invitation for loss or theft. Careful thought of financial cost and emotional attachment help determine whether to risk damage and grief if an item vanishes.

EXAMPLE: Shows resident and employee frustration when an administrator ignores theft.

Mrs. Dawson and Mother shared the same dining room table, a common background in food preparation and work experience. Mrs. Dawson's family restaurant served as the community's premier eatery for thirty years. Mother worked the same years in a school cafeteria and bowling alley grill. Each nursing home meal served to their table of four evoked a serious discussion of the food's quality and presentation.

Mother discussed food service logically and authoritatively in spite of her dementia. Mrs. Dawson said she appreciated the dining room conversations with Mother because, "She knows how good food is cooked and served. I don't think the rest of these people even know what they're eating."

A sound friendship developed even though Mrs. Dawson recognized Mother's limitations. She sympathized when Mother's glitzy, red beaded coin purse disappeared over the Thanksgiving weekend. The loss became a tearful upset for Mother even though it was inexpensive and contained only a few coins and a dollar bill.

Mr. Evans, the nursing home administrator, reminded me, "Mrs. Vance is very forgetful, she probably left it somewhere and another resident just picked it up and carried it off. I'll tell staff to be on the lookout." It did not return. Mother became more emotional as she ruminated over the loss.

I found a garish, flaming red, long haired, faux fur replacement about the size of an envelope. Mother got the message, "That thing will be hard for me to lose." She was happy with the coins and dollar bills tucked inside. Mrs. Dawson boosted Mother's spirit by adding a ten-dollar bill, her first Christmas present.

The facility's Christmas cheer did nothing to relieve another tearful breakdown when the bills disappeared three days later. The nursing staff routed me to the director of nursing who sent me to Mr. Evans with my theft report. I concluded theft because the purse was still in its place in the bedside stand.

Mr. Evans offered sympathy and a possibility. "Mrs. Vance probably gave the money to another resident and just doesn't remember. She's very generous, you know."

After voicing her dismay, Mrs. Dawson placed another ten-dollar bill in the red fuzzy coin purse. "Just another Christmas present," she said.

The bill disappeared the same night although the purse was spared. Mother's roommate, Vera, reminded me, "They're in here every night pilfering through our things."

Mr. Evans was too busy to talk with me so I began asking staff members if there were other thefts. Their shrugged shoulders and evasive body language was not surprising. Finally the frustrated charge nurse said, "You just have to talk to the administrator."

Undeterred, Mrs. Dawson placed a twenty-dollar bill in the red purse. Mother explained sadly, "Said she's just fixing stolen presents." Three days later I found Mother sitting on her bedside in an angry, rebellious mood. The entire purse was gone. Her trembling, tearful request was clear, "Please get me out of this hell hole. I need to go home to my friends."

Mr. Evans was still busy. I began asking visitors if their loved ones had problems with theft. The social worker appeared quickly to remind me of my signature on the Release of Responsibility Form.

His usually cavalier personality became sternly authoritative. "We will allow you to purchase a safe for Mrs. Vance's room. Only she will have the key or combination then she will always have control of her possessions."

"Oscar," I asked, "How can Mother remember a combination or keep up with a key? How does she use any kind of lock when she can't see well enough to find it and then her arthritic hands won't turn it?"

"Well, that's our solution," he retorted.

"Oscar," I probed, "where would you put a safe in this room every inch is taken up?"

"Oh, you can put one on top of the bedside stand."

"I think a safe on top of this flimsy furniture is unsafe. It might fall off and hurt somebody if they bump into it. The weight of a safe heavy enough to prevent someone from carrying it off would collapse this bedside stand. We just can't do that," I reasoned.

His stiff stance, clenched jaw and clipboard gripped tightly against his chest indicated resolve to deliver the boss's message. "Then you're responsible."

As he turned to leave I asked, "Does anyone ever just call the law?"

"Law enforcement can't help with confused, forgetful residents," he snorted and stomped away.

Later in the afternoon a young nursing assistant delivered clean linen and quietly confided, "They know who stole Mrs. Vance's money, everybody knows, they just won't do anything. She's not the only resident with things missing. Last week I cashed my paycheck at lunch and the cash was gone from my purse when I got off work. I told Mr. Evans right then. He could've done something—she was still on the clock. He just told me, 'don't bring cash to work.'" Her trembling voice verified the mother's sorrow, "Now I don't know how I'll get my kids Christmas presents."

Mother found the furry purse in her bedside stand the next day. Shaking it upside down to highlight its emptiness she lamented, "They took my last penny." The return was a reminder of the theft accompanied by repetitive, tearful pleadings "just let me go home, just let me go home."

The following day Mother proudly called my attention to a gorgeous new red blouse hanging prominently in her closet. Vera explained, "Mrs. Dawson went Christmas shopping with her daughter and bought that present for Mrs. Vance. I think she's given up on money presents."

Mother proudly wore the new blouse to the Christmas party that evening. The gift exchange brought glee. She received a pleasing collection of skin and body products. A lime colored felt bag held the toiletries. The trendy brand name was inscribed in rhinestones across the top.

Mother took great care to tuck her treasure into the tight space between her bed and the bedside stand . . . considering it safe even though difficult to retrieve. Then she kicked it further into the gap—all the way to the wall for good measure.

Her efforts were wasted. The next afternoon I found Mother and Vera consumed by a nervous, angry discussion. "The S.O.B.s found it," Mother shouted, pointing to the bag lying on her bed. "Well, they did leave me that one little bottle. Why didn't they just take the whole thing?"

Vera anxiously interjected, "I heard them over there last night but I was afraid to yell. You know they have ways of getting even.

They just quit answering your light or won't take you to the bathroom on time. Everybody was at the party last night so they knew who got good gifts."

As Vera trembled I tried to reassure her. "Vera, you did the right thing. I'll take care of this. Just be sure your sister takes everything you really don't need back home."

I attempted to divert Mother's attention. "You know what Daddy always said 'if somebody steals something they must need it worse than you.' Besides, you don't need all that sweet smelling stuff."

"What the hell do you mean? I might be looking for a man," she roared. We all chuckled. Her refrain indicated return to a familiar place in her mind, "Honey, get me out of here, I need to go back home with my friends."

My complaint to Mr. Evans drew his scripted, corporate response denying the possibility of employee theft. His echo seemed an insult to the intelligence of residents, their families and his employees. I resolutely decided to compile the dates and value of each theft and call the sheriff.

Mother was hospitalized the next day. She fell while serving coffee to her fellow diners. Mrs. Dawson explained, "Mrs. Vance wanted us to have hot coffee." She perceived food and coffee on the unattended serving cart was getting cold.

A sheriff's report was never filed. The thefts became trivial as Mother's hospitalization dominated my time and energy. Thus, Mr. Evans was able to forget and bury any trace of our theft complaints.

EXAMPLE: How one resident adjusted to theft.

The foyer's after-supper gathering always provided amusement and an update on the day's activities—no need to ask questions, just listen. Seats were limited to one hard bench but the small space always became congested with parked wheelchairs and rolling walkers with built-in seats. Some ladies just sauntered through to catch up on the day's happenings. Men kept their distance.

Residents enjoyed the entertainment offered by visitors entering and leaving the foyer. The building's only entrance gave them a chance to greet visitors and report anything new to residents' families. After visitors gingerly weaved through the gaggle and disappeared into the building, residents often discussed their attire.

I slipped onto the bench beside Mother, a seat almost hidden by an oversized, fake fern. As one entrant disappeared Mother said, "I sure like those red shoes she had on. Wish I had a pair."

"Well, that's Joe's daughter. She can afford good shoes and a different pair every day. I hear he's turned the ranch over to her," Olga quipped as she adjusted the colorful lap blanket covering her legs. The oversized wheelchair barely accommodated her girth.

"My red shoes got stolen," Olga mentioned casually.

"What kind of shoes?" Lula, a former bank teller queried.

"Red patent dancing shoes. Wish I could go dancing again." Olga stared sentimentally into the sunset beaming through the front door's full-length glass.

"Why would somebody steal old shoes?" Mother wondered aloud.

"Because she wanted to go dancing, but she brought 'em back. Yep, they're back in my closet."

Lula asked the question rolling in my head. "How could somebody steal 'em if they're in your closet?"

"I never missed 'em. Just saw 'em sitting there one day covered in fresh mud."

Mother became engaged, "When did this happen?"

"The last time it rained. Wasn't that last spring? Anyway, I wasn't walking in the mud. Haven't had on shoes in years . . . can't even stand up." Olga leaned forward pulling up the coverlet to reveal swollen feet. She nodded toward bulky socks stretched over arthritic deformities. "All I can get on now," she sighed, as if confirming footwear limitations to herself.

Jesse, the aged schoolteacher, slipped her svelte rolling walker closer into the group, sat down on its convenient seat and asked, "Who did it?"

"Just figure it out for yourself. Only one person works here with feet as big as mine. Who wears a size twelve, triple D?" The ladies immersed themselves in deep thought.

After several minutes Mother asked, "Did you tell anybody?"

Olga stared out the front door into approaching darkness before growing philosophical. "No, I didn't say anything because I like her and she takes good care of me. She's big and strong. She lifts me into bed easy, doesn't hurt. Wish she'd asked. She can borrow my shoes anytime but I'd want her to clean the mud off next time. Go look at 'em. The mud's still there."

A nursing assistant approached quietly, "Are you ready for bed Olga? I can help you now."

"Oh yes, Janie, I'm ready anytime you can help me. You get me in bed so easy," Olga replied.

Janie planted her feet solidly on the floor as if to gain traction then leaned into the handles of the extra wide wheelchair. They slipped down the hall as all eyes concentrated on Janie's feet. The ladies sat silently for several minutes before meandering off to bed without comment.

EXAMPLE: Portrays a resident's suspicions of theft.

Mrs. Garcia proudly showed her new handbag to anyone entering the room. The birthday present from her son conveyed expensive elegance with its soft brown leather and tasteful mother-of-pearl handle. She decided not to use the purse but put it away for Easter.

Turmoil ensued within a few days when Mrs. Garcia reported her purse stolen. She paced the halls, wringing her hands and asking everyone in sight, "Why would anybody steal an old woman's purse?" The staff looked in the other resident's rooms and searched the building.

The administrator apologized and accurately explained to Mrs. Garcia's son, "We don't have theft in this building." The administrator's message to staff was stern and non-forgiving, "If we can't find that purse, somebody stole it." The facility-wide search she ordered disrupted schedules and added to the workload without finding the purse.

The patient son asked about the missing purse on each visit. Staff discussed the perplexing situation often.

They rejected the administrator's idea of a thief in their midst. After working together for many years they knew each other well.

Housekeeping's faithful rotation for deep cleaning rooms required ladders to open the tight compartments wedged between the closet tops and ceiling. Neither staff nor residents used the spaces because the seven-foot-high handles were out of reach.

Dusting the space in Mrs. Garcia's room proved to be a godsend when the housekeeper discovered her purse thrown to the back of the compartment a week before Easter.

A relieved staff speculated about how the 5' 2" resident managed to hide her purse in the impossible space. "Probably climbed up on a chair and tossed it up there—a wonder she didn't fall and kill herself," her son concluded.

Mrs. Garcia did not remember hiding the purse. She did remember accusing the staff of "robbing a poor, helpless old lady." Guilt emerged. Another tearful, hand-wringing saga erupted with days of apologizing for her false accusations.

All seemed well by Easter Sunday. She swaggered out to church conspicuously swinging the purse. Pride in the faithful son escorting her added to her pleasure. His subtle wink and nod to staff relayed a silent "thank you" and his own relief.

Chapter 19

LAUNDRY

Personal laundry service is included in the nursing home's daily room rate. Turnaround and individualized attention for personal clothing varies significantly between facilities.

A visit to the laundry can be beneficial toward understanding its role in overall building operations and residents' comfort level. Handling of dirty clothing and linen presents huge challenges related to infections, odors, adequate linen supplies for nursing staff and processing individual clothing. Imagine folding underwear and matching socks for two hundred residents. When wash, dry, fold and hanging are complete, laundry staff faces the task of returning each piece of clothing to the correct closet or drawer. This occurs only after linen closets have been restocked for the nursing staff.

The laundry is usually detached from the main building due to the risk of explosion and fire. The heat produced by massive industrial dryers renders air conditioning useless. Large exhaust fans provide some relief in summer, but it is not unusual for temperatures inside the laundry to exceed an outside temperature of 100 degrees.

Laundry staff may have the most difficult and thankless job in the facility. They are minimally staffed and expected to keep clean linen and clothing flowing even when some machines are awaiting repair, which is quite often in some buildings.

Each new resident's responsible party would do well to visit with the laundry supervisor soon after admission. Ask their opinion about how to mark clothing and what kind of clothing works best for the laundry. Thus, you will establish a connection between the new resident and their clothing. The contact will serve you well if problems arise.

You will find additional insight in the BE AWARE and BEWARE sections below. EXAMPLES of laundry quandaries follow.

BE AWARE

- Even within a facility boasting good laundry services there will be daily variations from good to bad service.
- Personal clothing is collected in fifty-five-gallon roll-around barrels and thrown with the other residents clothing into huge institutional washers.
- There is no attempt to separate fine delicates from heavy denim or light soiled from heavy soiled.
- Do not expect any attention to stain removal or any selective care.
- The industrial size dryers are harsh and you must expect the hottest of temperatures.
- The high dryer temperatures do assure some degree of organism death and thwart the transmission of disease through personal clothing.
- Facility linen is of necessity given priority over personal clothing because only a few buildings have enough sheets, towels, washcloths and padding to assure availability beyond an eight-hour shift.

BEWARE
- All clothing needs to be marked with the resident's last name. You would do well to mark it yourself with a permanent marker to ensure an inside, inconspicuous spot visible only to laundry personnel. Otherwise, you may find the family name emblazoned across the back of a blouse, waistband or the top of socks.
- Residents' personal laundry can be collected for their family to launder. This process can be frustrating if staff fails to deposit clothing in your marked "Personal Laundry" basket in the room.
- Personal clothing disappears during the laundry cycle. Questions of theft abound and are sometimes warranted. Often the explanation is just delivery to the wrong room or slow turnaround in the laundry.
- If you find yourself in a particularly bad laundry situation you may need to bring clothing for special occasions and take it back with you the same day. Sometimes you can depend upon a watchful nurse or nursing assistant to collect the clothes for you at day's end.

EXAMPLE: How one resident's laundry woes may be an indication of larger problems.

"Please come talk to Mrs. Erwin's daughter. She's livid." The nurse summoned me from another unit and she needed to say no more. As weekend nurse manager for the building, I recalled many conversations with the daughter. All were related to the laundry.

"Why can't they just put her dirty clothes in the basket? It's right there, they must be able to see it!" She was referring to a collection basket for her mother's laundry, clearly marked and very visible. She preferred laundering her mother's clothing and faithfully collected the contents every few days. Often the basket contained only a few pieces of clothing or nothing. "You know they tear up her pretty clothes or they never get back when they end up in the laundry," the daughter pleaded.

My discussions with the nursing assistants always elicited a repetitive answer. "Ms. Frances, the regulars know about Mrs. Erwin's clothes but new hires and aides pulled from other units just throw everything in the laundry barrels; it's easier and faster."

I remembered talking with laundry personnel and requesting, "Please watch for Mrs. Erwin's clothing when it comes through." The only reply was an exasperated nod from the laundry supervisor. With half her washing capacity awaiting repair and over two hundred residents in-house, I understood.

The daughter and I spent previous Saturdays in the laundry, going through piles of unfolded personal clothing. We never retrieved anything belonging to Mrs. Erwin.

I arrived at the nurse's station to find the daughter near tears. "Mother has new clothes, good clothes, missing. Look, her clothes basket's empty." She waved the empty basket as she took a more cynical tone. "But, this morning Mother had on her top that's been missing for eighteen months. Now if they would just find the missing bottom!"

I began sympathetic apologies only to be interrupted, "It's hopeless. I give up. I do appreciate you trying to help me." Her defeat and disappointment were evident as she walked away with the empty clothes basket.

I was relieved that she did not request to search the laundry today. Earlier I investigated complaints of bad odors from the building's south wing and followed my nose to twenty-three overflowing barrels of putrid linen and clothing outside the laundry. The frazzled laundry supervisor told me, "I've had a washer down for a week and the personal clothes just keep stacking up. I'll never be able to get some of them clean, they're just rotting in the sun."

I hoped the gentle breeze would shift giving the south wing relief from the nauseous smell. I asked housekeeping to be generous with their aerosol deodorizers then braced for more trouble; one nurse had already informed me, "We're out of linen barrels, they're all stacked up in the laundry."

There would be no weekend washer repairs. Several changes in ownership, management and bankruptcies resulted in years of uncollectible invoices throughout the city. Any local service or purchase required prepayment. The facility's local bank account had no money, only a few dollars in petty cash and the credit card had been confiscated by the out-of-state corporate office. These executives were less than helpful in resolving our administrator's dilemma. Their instructions: "Find somebody who *will* invoice the job." The merits of replacing the aged, often out-of-service washer were never considered.

EXAMPLE: Laundry problems complicated by theft and staffing limitations.

Laundry at Mother's first nursing home was routine with a dependable turnaround of one to three days. Occasional rips and accidental bleaching were always explained to mother's satisfaction.

The second nursing home's laundry presented perpetual problems. Lost outer garments were usually retrieved after complaints, but her new, expensive underwear disappeared forever. Only one or two pieces out of a dozen placed in circulation would ever make it back to mother's drawer. Old, worn, ragged underwear came back with regularity. Some didn't belong to Mother but seemed to be a replacement for the missing. Talks with the laundry supervisor, Bella, elicited my sympathy. She made a real effort to watch for Mother's distinctive panties and bras but told me, "It's really hard to know what goes on after I leave in the afternoon. I

LAUNDRY

can't say much because we need help so bad." Complaints to the nursing home administrator only directed me back to Bella.

After several months of frustration, Bella suggested we place Mother's underwear in a mesh bag, she would watch for the bag. The chore of underwear collection kept Mother busy for two laundry cycles until the bag disappeared leaving her distraught again.

Mother's roommate, Vera, cautioned, "Don't put anything nice in that laundry. You'll never see it again. There's nothing but a bunch of thieves out there."

My sister took care of Mother's wardrobe, I told her, "Just send plain, simple, inexpensive underwear." She wasn't helpful and continued to send delicate, soft panties and expensive bras because, "That's what Mother likes."

Mother became fixated on her problem. She did not want to wear ugly, torn underwear. After one tearful episode she solved the problem to her satisfaction by washing her underwear in the bathroom sink.

I found panties and bras hanging from the towel rack dripping abundant water on the floor in addition to water splattered over the bathroom. The hand-soap dispenser was empty but soapy bubbles ran down the wall.

Sitting on the bed, arms crossed, sleeves wet to the elbows, Mother linked herself to the mess. "Don't need that thievin' laundry, can still wash my own drawers."

"I know you can Mother, but I'm worried about somebody slipping in this water. You've already told me I can shoot you if you break a leg but what about Vera? We can't shoot her." Any rebuke would only cause anxiety.

Vera's comment was more helpful, "Mrs. Vance, you pay this place good money. Make 'em get your clothes right."

This time Bella suggested placing only one set of new underwear into the laundry cycle every few weeks, "It's easier for me to watch one new bra and panty than keep up with six new ones in the same week. After a couple of runs through the laundry nobody wants them anyway."

I followed her advice and brought one pair of new underwear as others became worn and faded. The situation improved although never resolved completely, Mother was satisfied. She told Vera, "We got that laundry straight."

CHAPTER 20

HOLIDAYS AND GIFTS

Holidays, anniversaries, birthdays and special occasions present questions and dilemmas about the right gifts for nursing home residents. Of utmost importance are the mental and physical capabilities of the resident.

Are they alert, talkative, interested in their surroundings or perhaps confused, withdrawn or unable to communicate? Physical status means a great deal: can the resident get around the nursing home without assistance or do they need help; are they busy with nursing home activities or do they prefer solitude; are they confined to the bed or a recliner?

There are substantial limitations within the nursing home; space is minimal, safety must prevail, spread of infections is always a concern, pest control problems never end. Each facility may have additional concerns and restrictions.

If you haven't seen the resident for a while there is the possibility that their condition has changed since your last contact. A call to someone who sees them frequently might be helpful, whether a family member, nurse or activities director. Hopefully, you will find a staff member willing to help by asking, "What does Julie need, what would she enjoy?" Just remember, they cannot give you specific information about the resident's medical or physical condition.

Suggestions are listed in BE AWARE, cautions appear in BEWARE and EXAMPLES follow.

BE AWARE
- Cards and letters are a great gift especially when spread across the entire year. A positive update about old friends and yourself is uplifting. Just leave out the bad news on which residents tend to ruminate for days. The activities department and volunteers will read notes and letters to residents who need help. Never underestimate the value of such reading to residents who seem totally withdrawn or even comatose.

- Food should be in tight containers of tin or plastic. No glass, it presents dangers with breakage. Individual wrapping of each treat is best to avoid contamination by multiple hands. Alert residents enjoy having singly wrapped mints and hard candies to offer the staff. Special diets such as diabetic, low salt and fluid restrictions should always be considered. Never leave food at the bedside of a resident with swallowing problems.
- Toiletries are best limited to simple skin moisturizers, lotions and shaving cream. A bottle of lotion sitting at the bedside is a convenience for caretakers and enjoyed by the resident. Low fragrance is preferred. Avoid powders including talcum. They can be inhaled and also cause acidic reactions on the skin.
- Comfortable clothing is always welcome by residents and staff. Pull-on soft, cotton sweatpants and tops lead the list for men and women. Hooded tops provide extra warmth around the neck. The bright colors available can be used for mix and match. They launder well and are easily pulled on and off by staff. A simple neck scarf can add a personal touch.
    1. Men enjoy flannel shirts year round.
    2. Avoid frills and delicate materials especially in undergarments, they will never survive the laundry.
    3. Spare the staff and resident pullover nightgowns. Pulling them on and off is uncomfortable and time consuming.
    4. For men, soft cotton pajamas with elastic waistbands and pullover tops provide comfort and ease of changing.
    5. Front or back openings from neck to hem facilitate quick changes, which often occur in the middle of the night underneath a cold air conditioning vent.
    6. For residents confined to the bed or a recliner full back opening garments should be your only consideration. Soft cottons and fleece are always the preferred materials.
    7. Keep buttons, zippers and fasteners at a minimum. They are difficult for residents to manage, time consuming for staff and subject to damage in the laundry.
    8. Most nursing homes host independent vendors who offer a selection of beautiful, comfortable resident clothing for purchase once or twice annually. Check with the activity director for their next visit or contact information.

- Fleece blankets are a godsend providing warmth and cozy comfort. Their lightweight avoids any pressure on the skin. They launder well and are available in a variety of sizes.
- Newspapers are scarce at nursing homes. Consider an annual subscription to the resident's favorite newspaper. Most enjoy their hometown paper even though they may be dislocated and many miles away. Some prefer the nearest metro and a few even the Wall Street Journal. Most importantly a newspaper is delivered to them personally.
- Plants present problems with dirt contamination, spilled water and space limitations. Only a few residents are able to care for even a small plant so they should be avoided. Nevertheless, seasonal plants such as poinsettias and Easter lilies can brighten resident rooms for a few weeks.
- Cushions are a serviceable gift offering comfort for the resident who spends much of the day sitting.
    1. Sizes fitting into a regular pillowcase are convenient for staff.
    2. Soft fiber filling with cotton covers are easily laundered and soft.
    3. Foam cushions may not be allowed due to flammability. They are also difficult to sanitize.
    4. Avoid vinyl covers, which tend to become hard and non-flexible. They are non-porous causing sweating and moisture collection. A cleansing wipe down is easy but often overlooked.
    5. Gel cushions provide the best pressure reductions for residents sitting for long periods.
- Medical equipment can provide comfort, convenience and independence for nursing home residents. Nursing homes are expected to provide any equipment residents need. Medicare and Medicaid will not pay for personal equipment after admission to a nursing home because the daily room rate paid by Medicare and Medicaid is calculated to include such equipment. The nursing home is not required to assign equipment to individual residents. Typically, they just keep an inventory available for everyone to use. Since residents share the same equipment, availability may be limited or involve waiting while staff scrambles to locate a walker or wheelchair.

In most nursing homes the bottom-line price for the basic models dictates their selection. Ease of use, functionality and updated features are rarely considered. However, private gifting provides endless possibilities. What better use of personal resources for a resident in the Medicaid spend down situation? When no longer needed, the equipment can be donated for a charitable tax deduction.

1. Walkers provide safety and independence for residents and are inexpensive. Consider a plain or rolling walker or one of the sleek models with a seat and hand brakes. The nursing home's physical therapist can help you decide on the appropriate walker.
2. Wheelchair availability and condition are never assured in the nursing home unless residents own their own. Purchased wheelchairs are customized to the resident's height, weight and attachment needs such as headrest, leg and foot supports. Why not an electric wheelchair to enhance the everyday pleasure of an alert resident who enjoys activities throughout the nursing home?
3. Mattresses are the greatest gift of all. Nursing home mattresses are often uncomfortable but rarely seen or discussed. Visitors usually see the mattress covered and are not aware of the stains, sinks and weaknesses of too many years' use. If a visual examination passes muster, try lying down on the mattress. Would you like to spend eight to twenty-four hours in succession on this mattress? State-of-the-art foam mattresses provide comfort, restful sleep and rejuvenation.
4. Why not an electric bed if your loved one's facility is still using manual (hand-cranked) beds? A good electric bed provides comfortable positioning, safety, convenience and a degree of independence at a mere touch of a button. Half-length side-rails provide residents a handgrip for turning in bed and stable support to sit on the bedside or stand up. Large color-coded controls embedded in the rails allow even a weak, arthritic resident to control the bed's contour with a light touch. Independently changing the head elevation or moving the entire bed to lounge chair position provides freedom

and self-control for the resident and saves staff time and work. Stylish models are available to match any bedroom or nursing home décor and bear no resemblance to a hospital bed.
5. Consider the everlasting pleasure of a new mattress delivered atop a new electric bed directly to your loved one.

BEWARE
- The most enjoyable holiday outings are best planned with the resident's comfort and limitations in mind. Restaurant dining remains high on the list. The trip can be difficult and stressful for one resident although pleasurable for another.
- Frequent visitors seem to understand their loved ones' limitations and make pragmatic decisions about activities outside the facility. They often realize that a special meal within a quiet place in the building or special dining room arrangements result in less stress and more pleasant holidays for all concerned.
- Staffing limits demand ample notification for special requests—specific clothing and pick-up times—of at least twenty-four hours.
- Gifts to residents in special care units (Alzheimer's, memory care, secure and locked areas) require individual consideration depending upon the stage of the resident's dementia. Check with staff or family prior to visiting or sending gifts.
- Don't even consider expensive jewelry. Theft, loss and unexplained disappearances are rampant in many nursing homes. The jewelry lover can enjoy inexpensive, easily replaced costume jewelry without the angst of a loss. The nursing home will not be responsible for any losses.
- Expensive or fine clothing is a bad choice. Nursing home laundries are not staffed or equipped to provide the special care these garments require. Even underwear may never find its way back to your resident.
- Expensive toiletries, bath products and lotions are impractical and often disappear before the resident has a chance to use or enjoy the gift.
- Everything needs to be marked. The preferred method is a permanent marker with the resident's last name. Staff is too

busy to track down ownership of unmarked personal articles. Family members, activities personnel and laundry staff will help with marking although it's far more practical to mark the gift before it's delivered.

EXAMPLE: A holiday outing which seems to have misplaced intent - it focused on the family member rather than the resident.

Visits peak on Mother's Day. Family members flood the building often giving the appearance of performing a duty rather than looking forward to a pleasing experience. Residents cannot ignore the increased traffic. Staff faces a barrage of special requests. Lunch outside the facility dominates family plans. Those unfamiliar with facility routine often arrive unannounced with new attire and expectations of immediate help; subsequent delays lead to demands staff cannot fulfill, then add stress and discomfort for Mother.

I recall the daughter who showed up to take her mother out to lunch, but demanded the nurse do something about her mother's black eye. In the Mother's presence, she said, "I can't take her anywhere looking like this!" The daughter rarely visited and notification of a fall and resultant shiner a week earlier meant little to her at the time. The resident's nurse of many months met the daughter for the first time, explained the black eye again and observed their departure for the restaurant. The petite, meticulously dressed resident looked despondent as she walked through the lobby with her angry daughter.

Her nurse asked, "Why bother?"

EXAMPLE: How a gift can face resistance from a facility's administrator even though previously discussed and approved by the administrator.

Mother's new electric bed sat at the end of the hallway for several days. We faced unexpected resistance after its delivery. The first hurdle was the administrator's concern that other residents would expect the same kind of bed, but paid for by the facility. Next, questions of safety arose, even though it was tagged with an official universal safety sticker and arrived new from the manufacturer. Then we waited a few more days for the maintenance man to check the bed's operation for safety issues. Then the family became responsible for obtaining a physician's order for the bed!

After all the conditions were satisfied, the administrator would not allow facility staff to move the bed into Mother's room. He said, "They do not have the time and the facility would be liable if they damaged the bed."

Later that evening, after office hours and the administrator's departure, I summoned Mother's grandsons to make the switch. She mastered the simple controls within a few minutes and began enjoying all the comforts of a new bed and mattress.

We left the old bed as a replacement at the end of hall. When I returned the next day the hallway was clear. No one from administration mentioned the bed again, but nursing assistants commented often on the convenience for them. When Mother died we left the bed for her roommate and best friend. She enjoyed it as much as Mother.

EXAMPLE: The value of a newspaper.

A colleague from my company's medical sales division once told me about a nursing home encounter.

As he entered a facility the resident in a nearby wheelchair caught his eye. The "old man" as he described him, looked a mess: wrinkled clothes, days old food stains on his shirt, unshaven, disheveled white hair. Appearance aside, his demeanor corresponded to that of a corporate boardroom. He sat upright. Piercing eyes stared over the top of reading glasses as he sized up the visitor, but he said nothing. His authoritative glare seemed to demand recognition.

The young salesman responded, "Good morning, Sir."

The gentleman answered with the trace of a nod, then returned to his newspaper.

My friend elaborated, "He was working the crossword puzzle with a pen . . . not a pencil, but an ink pen! Furthermore, it was the Wall Street Journal and he was almost finished! There was somebody home."

"There usually is," I answered.

References

CUSHION and MATTRESS COVERS: Vinyl retains moisture and body heat on its surface, thus increasing the risk of skin rashes and sores. Additionally, vinyl coverings are harder than the pressure reduction materials inside cushions and mattresses, therefore, a barrier between the resident and the therapeutic effects of the cushions and mattresses. Alternatives are soft, loose, synthetic fabric covers that stretch to body contours, resist moisture and allow air movement.

ELECTRIC BEDS: Long-term-care electric beds are engineered to accommodate nursing home residents' needs—safety, comfort and convenience. Safety: choices of lowering to within a few inches of the floor or waist height for staff, and half siderails with entrapment prevention. Comfort: readily adjusted therapeutic positioning for medical conditions and automatic contours to assist with posture. Convenience: large color-coded controls require only a soft touch (gnarled, stiff fingers manage controls with a tap) to adjust their own positioning, including lounge chair sitting.

Controls for electric beds may be attached to an electrical cord like a pendant or mounted in the bed siderails. Full length siderails are disappearing from newer models due to safety issues . . . their history of resident injuries. Beds must meet International Electrotechnical Committee (IEC) standards in order to comply with the nursing home's life safety standards. Beds are sold by a plethora of manufacturers, distributors and medical equipment retail stores. The best nursing home beds are free of bells and whistles and provide simplicity of operation, durability, warranty and service. One example: http://www.adaptivespecialties.com/hill-rom-resident-ltc.aspx

More facilities are purchasing electric beds because they are a requirement for some private insurance contracts. Many insurers will not sign a contract unless the nursing home provides electric beds for their patients leaving the hospital for skilled nursing care. However, facilities are less likely to provide electric beds for the remainder of their residents.

CHAPTER 21
ADVOCACY

Although the burden of physical care is relieved by nursing home admission, a heavier load may be the realization that you are still the best one to guide care, furthermore your guidance must fit within institutional policies. Barriers to a resident's individual interests never end. Advocacy (support) for your loved one can be exhausting and the best survival tactic may be to understand and choose your battles. The squeaky wheel approach garners immediate attention, but everyone's interests are best served by lasting solutions.

The best advocacy is the resident's self-promotion if they are alert and competent, but self-advocates still need family or responsible party backup during controversial periods. Indeed, everyone needs support for the journey through the nursing home industry's maze. During my nursing home career, I found one distinguishing trait among effective advocates - they genuinely care about the resident. Among them are spouses, adult children and friends who visit consistently and quietly. Staff recognizes these caring advocates and understands their easiest path is to work *with* such a spokesperson.

Successful advocates exhibit perseverance, patience and a willingness to learn the workings and mindset of the facility. The most effective advocacy is not unending demands but consistent, reasonable expectations. Unreasonable hassles may secure immediate action, but limited change. For example, staff may interrupt their schedule to cool down immediate demands; "I need mother's hair combed now!" But this does not assure her hair will be combed when you are not there.

Nursing home advocacy presents itself in many forms; often quiet, unseen moments become significant. Consider each facility a community of families, visitors, staff and residents. In a nursing home this network provides an endless source of oversight for each resident's care. Be prepared! You may develop warm attachments to roommates and other residents you encounter throughout the facility.

This familiarity leads to your own obligation to make staff aware when these residents need attention.

Occasional visitors also serve an important role in advocacy. Sometimes just their presence in the building reminds staff of responsibilities and moves them to take care of residents' needs a little quicker. It is important for visitors to find a staff member when observing something awry with any resident. Perhaps an incontinent episode needs attention, a resident is slipping out of their wheelchair, someone is asking for a drink, a resident is complaining of pain or is anxious and asking for help. Consider it your responsibility to tell staff of immediate problems you see while in the building.

The person listed as the responsible party carries the most influence over resident care and will be the only person capable of changes in the resident's *care plan*. Family members not designated as the responsible party have influence over *routine* care, schedules and activities if there is no conflict with the care plan. Non-family visitors play an important role in assuring that reasonable care is being provided.

Be prepared for upending of agreements and understandings during changes in facility ownership and personnel which occurs all too often in nursing homes. Rest assured, your acquired knowledge, expertise and contacts within the facility position you as an effective negotiator when upheavals occur.

Remember, people do not give up individual rights upon entering a nursing home, especially police reports and protection.

The BE AWARE and BEWARE sections provide more insight and suggestions. EXAMPLES follow.

BE AWARE
There are Ten Commandments of Advocacy. This approach is not foolproof, but it does provide shrewd insight beginning on admission day.
1. Visit on all shifts in order to learn personnel and routine. You learn a lot by asking staff concerned questions; "What time did you come to work?" "You look really busy today." Response to such questions will often include additional bits of information you may need later such as short staffing. You will also learn which employees care about residents and who couldn't care less.

2. Identify two or three nurses who seem to care about your resident. Nurses on different shifts are preferable because you will need their help later, you can expect problems on all shifts.
3. Find two or three nurse's aides (CNAs) who show sympathy and gentle attention to your resident. You will need to spread these out over all shifts also.
4. Housekeeping and maintenance are usually thankless jobs. Acknowledge the presence of the housekeeper and maintenance man when you see them in the hall. Thank them when they are working in the room . . . you will need favors later and they have a choice of which projects to do first or maybe just delay.
5. Thank laundry personnel when they deliver clean clothing to the room and ask their opinion about simple things; "What kind of fabrics are the easiest for you to run through the laundry?" You may face laundry problems and these conversations will help you understand and deal with lost or damaged clothing.
6. Attendance at meetings and gatherings will send staff a message of involvement in your resident's care. Additionally, get-togethers provide opportunities to meet and network with other families.
7. Visit at meal times: it's your chance to check the quality of food and amount of servings. The evening meal is important. Some facilities save on food costs by scant servings and menu changes for the evening meal where there is less scrutiny. Staffing is often inadequate at the evening meal resulting in residents without feeding help and cold food.
8. Offer to help staff when you can: changing linen, pushing wheelchairs to the dining room and activities, assisting your loved one to the bathroom or to walk in the hall as part of their activity schedule. These gestures assure staff of your sincerity.
9. As soon as you find glitches in your resident's care begin the process of correcting the trouble. For non-nursing problems start with the responsible department head such as laundry, kitchen, activities, or social worker. "Mother doesn't like carrots; could you arrange a substitute?" "She loves bingo, could you include her?" Go to the facility administrator only when you cannot resolve the issue with a department head.
10. For nursing problems the best approach is discussion with the nurse's aides and nurses directly involved in your loved one's

care. Give these caregivers an opportunity to solve your problem before moving up the chain of command to the director of nurses or the administrator. "Mother keeps complaining that the hallway is cold. Could you remind her to put on a sweater before she leaves her room?"

Best results for your resident are obtained by utilizing multiple resources:
- Attentive residents become expert at learning employees and routines, but still need an advocate for reinforcement; this role increases as residents age and become more vulnerable.
- Family members or the responsible party are the advocates carrying the most influence. The best supporters learn the rules of the road in spite of frustrating and tedious procedures.
- Residents' families often build alliances of oversight with each other. By establishing relationships they naturally check on each others' loved ones when in the facility. Reports from networking families deliver a wealth of information on how your resident is treated in your absence.
- Residents become friends and advocates for each other. They are especially conscientious in reminding staff of duties. "Where's Joe's 10 o'clock snack?" "Alice needs help in the bathroom!" "Somebody forgot Tom's knee brace!"
- Never underestimate a roommate's value, even a confused roommate. They spend more time with your resident than anyone else. Friendships develop, advocacy results and information is gleaned. Mother's experience is a good example: Mother complained of a sore hip confirmed by a bruise...she told me of falling during the night but the nurses denied a fall. When no employees were within earshot Mother's roommate said, "Mrs. Vance fell hard last night. Maybe she just fell out of bed or was going to the bathroom but everybody heard the furniture banging around. Juan and Valerie came in here and put her back to bed...had to pick her up...she couldn't even get up."
- Volunteers are also advocates. Appearances of church, civic and school groups incentivize staff to get residents dressed and ready for events in order to avoid complaints.

Structured programs within the facility afford organized support:
- The ombudsman program assigns a volunteer to each nursing home. This ombudsman is available to negotiate disputes between the facility and residents when they are unable to resolve disagreements on their own. Ombudsmen have no regulatory or supervisory authority. They are trained to understand residents' rights and nursing home operations. Their insight is helpful because your problem may be a recurrent one within the building. Ombudsmen are not able to solve every problem since their role is limited to mediation. However, they carry considerable influence with regulatory agencies. You will find their contact information on the bulletin board.
- Resident Council is an organization of alert residents who identify problems and offer suggestions for improvement. The group elects officers; their president will be interviewed during inspections so the groups suggestions cannot be totally ignored by management-especially near inspection times. The Resident Council addresses general operational concerns not individual resident complaints. Resident Councils *are* mandated by regulations. Families are usually excluded from Resident Council meetings.
- Family Council is a meeting of families with intentions of improving the nursing home at large. Safety, maintenance, staffing or any other environmental issues may be discussed but not individual resident complaints. Their good will is often co-opted into payment commitments for the same projects they are proposing, i.e., if the Family Council asks for a new awning over the patio, the facility management wrangles them into conducting a fundraiser to pay for it. Family Council is *not* mandated by regulations. Facilities are not obligated to offer any support, but most facilities find them helpful. The absence of a Family Council does not bode well for advocacy.
- Care plan meetings are a chance to have your advocacy requests recorded.
- Each nursing home has a medical director responsible for oversight of medical care within the facility. Staff, families and legal guardians have access to this physician if they feel medical treatment by the resident's personal physician is inadequate or

harmful. This is, of course, a dead end if the medical director and personal physician are one and the same. Such is often the case and there are no peer review options of medical directors.

After a few weeks you will have identified key points like conscientious personnel and problem areas within the building, maybe, staffing, cleanliness, meals. Now you are relieved of frequent visits and know to visit during problem times.

- Additionally, you will know which employees are dependable and attentive to residents. Talk with these employees and build relationships. You will be rewarded with information gleaned from casual conversations. Your loved one may not remember or choose to inform you of adverse situations occurring in your absence. Employees are more apt to offer information to family members they trust.
- Pick your complaints and issues wisely. Decide how much influence to expend on any difficulty; thus establishing yourself as a concerned advocate rather than you becoming the problem. For example, safety issues such as unanswered call lights require maneuvering up the chain of command to the administrators office if unresolved. An unfulfilled request to dress mother in her purple outfit every Sunday evening to watch "The Lawrence Welk Show" demands your common sense compromise.

Employees are rarely thanked. Consider the Golden Rule and treat them the way you want to be treated.

- Snacks delivered to the staff reinforces your appreciation for their work. Learn the schedules of the helpful staff and deliver on their workdays.
- Many families bring cakes, cookies and candies during holidays. Those delivered off-season are standouts, especially home cooked.
- Bring trays labeled for each shift otherwise all is devoured by the receiving shift.
- A bucket of chicken or a pizza delivered to the nurse's station by you is associated with your resident. Deliver when you know staff's work is difficult such as weekends.

- Spread out your meal deliveries on different days and different shifts. Use this tactic to acknowledge employees helpful to your resident.
- A treat or meal will not incentivize uncaring staff to provide more attention to your resident.

Long distance advocacy presents hurdles but there are options.
- Encourage family or friends in the area to visit often and report back to you.
- Call frequently to talk to the resident and staff. You can ascertain subtle changes during these conversations. Try to identify one or two nurses willing to impart information and ask to speak with them.
- Visit as often as possible but always unannounced.
- There are a few elder care businesses whose personnel visit and oversee senior citizens in all settings for a fee.
- Cameras mounted in resident rooms have proven to be controversial but enlightening for total care bed patients. Other residents spend most of their time off camera.

BEWARE
- Confrontation and complaints are the least effective form of advocacy but may be necessary. Never hesitate to notify the state inspectors if you are unable to resolve safety or health care issues. Examples are scalding hot tap water or failure to give medications correctly. Contact numbers are located in the resident rooms, nurses' station and bulletin board.
- Threatening legal action is usually fruitless. Most plaintiff attorneys are too unfamiliar with nursing homes to provide immediate relief, but corporate based facilities have their own string of lawyers ready to defend poor practices. Remember, the legal system moves very slowly and a resident can suffer real harm including death, while waiting.
- Residents may embellish or misinterpret situations. Remain objective thus avoiding manipulation by your resident. They can be stinkers.
- Physical or sexual abuse demands immediate notification of local law enforcement. Beyond your moral responsibility, many states consider observers an accomplice, subject to conviction

if not reported. You cannot depend upon facility personnel to report to authorities. It is your responsibility.
- Verbal abuse should be reported immediately to the administrator and state inspectors. After business hours there will be a designated supervisor in-house or a manager on call. Nurses should have these numbers.
- If you find yourself in a recurring cycle of negligent care, another nursing home may be your only solution.

EXAMPLE: A daughter's advocacy encounters roadblocks from her family, the physician, the nursing home and legal entanglements. The resident's worsening condition and the impasse created an emergent situation.

I received a frantic call from a friend. "Frances, they're killing my mother! What do I do?"

Ann had not visited her mother, Gloria, in a Missouri nursing home for several months. The descriptions of Gloria's physical condition seemed to warrant her hysteria. "She can barely talk, has infected sores on her legs, won't eat or drink anything. I think she's dehydrated. Mother wants to go to the hospital."

Family disagreements, belligerent facility staff and a manipulative mother complicated the grave situation. Ann and her brother had not spoken in years and he was now Mother's power of attorney. Nursing home personnel refused to give Ann any information on Gloria's condition stating that her power of attorney had instructed them not to do so. They refused to transfer her to the hospital because the power of attorney's written instructions included no transfer to any hospital—probably an advanced directive. In refusing to talk with Ann, the physician claimed he was following the power of attorney instructions.

Gloria's requests to go to the hospital were ignored even though she had not been determined incompetent. She requested Ann's help but shunned any discussion of changing legal arrangements.

After a twenty-four-hour impasse, I advised Ann, "Call the state inspectors and report neglect and abuse. That is the only option left. If you report any lesser violations they will take days or weeks to investigate."

With the arrival of state inspectors the next day, intravenous fluids with antibiotics were begun and increased staff attention resulted in physical improvement. However, this was only the beginning of a long slog of revisiting the same repetitive hurdles.

Ann's situation shines light on several problems detrimental to Gloria's comfort and health. Most important is a nursing home's willingness to dismiss a resident's rights i.e. her requests to go to the hospital. Gloria's physician is also the medical director and grateful for the facility's monthly income, he will not be found in opposition to any facility decisions. A dysfunctional family dynamic is contrary to Gloria's best interest and her controlling manipulation is contrary to her own well-being.

EXAMPLE: Advocacy in the absence of a family or responsible party.

Adult Protective Services (APS) knew little about the eighty-five-year-old they brought to our San Antonio nursing home. The agency visited his home after the public utilities reported they were shutting off power for non-payment in an elder's home. Subsequent investigation revealed no food or money but rooms full of magazines stacked to the ceiling.

Unkempt, thin and articulate the new resident announced, "I do not need to be here." A bit resistive yet well-mannered, he presented none of the usual behavior problems. Instead he deftly protested every move by staff. "Young lady, I do not need my blood pressure taken."

"Yes sir, I understand but it would help me a lot if I could take your blood pressure," the nurse's aide replied as the resident cupped his ear and leaned closer for better hearing.

"Okay ma'am, go right ahead but I don't need anything else."

"Well, Mr. Andrews, I'm going to bring you some lunch as soon as I get this blood pressure and I think I can find you an extra dessert, unless you don't eat sweets."

The stoic new resident remained aloof, "Yes ma'am, lunch would be appreciated since you have me incarcerated. I never turn down a dessert."

Soon after lunch a sharp dressed man attired in a business suit, stiffly starched white shirt, gold cufflinks and glossy shined shoes appeared at the nurse's station. He identified himself as John Andrews' next-door neighbor; the nurse directed him to the room at the end of a long hall.

Everyone on the hall heard the greeting. "Andrews, what the hell's going on over there? Those people from downtown are all over the neighborhood asking questions about you."

"Well, I've just got a damn mess," the new resident yelled as a thoughtful employee closed the door.

Before leaving the neighbor told staff that Mr. Andrews had been his neighbor for over twenty years. They talked over the fence but he hadn't noticed anything wrong . . . just hadn't seen him for a while. The neighbor assured staff he would find out details of the mess and locate his hearing aids. "You know he can't hear it thunder! Does he need anything else?"

Over the next few weeks the neighbor proved to be an ideal advocate and intermediary. He kept staff up to date; we learned of Mr. Andrew's obsession with Publisher's Clearinghouse Sweepstakes. He felt the more magazine subscriptions he bought the greater his chances of winning. All his savings and monthly income had been depleted for magazine purchases. Bills were unpaid and there was no money for groceries.

The neighbor negotiated with APS, the nursing home social worker, Meals on Wheels and other community resources for support if he returned home. He sought staff opinions about his neighbor's ability to care for himself and take medications correctly. All professionals involved in his care agreed on his possibility of returning home, if he stayed away from his previous obsession. The APS insisted upon a guardian type oversight for a while.

Mr. Andrews' neighbor agreed to be available but only after he employed his impressive business skills. He asked a nurse and social worker to conference in the resident's room where he informed him of his conditional help. "Andrews if you spend one cent on sweepstakes, I'm through, you end up right back here, incarcerated." The resident was quick to agree and the neighbor enjoyed some leverage with his nursing home witnesses. He later confided to staff, "I have no idea if this ultimatum will work."

The significance of this example is the objectivity of the advocate and his willingness to enlist staff's participation. The mutual respect and cooperation was a significant factor in the resident's return home.

EXAMPLE: A family advocate.

Mr. Johnson always picked up his mother at 9:00 a.m. sharp on Sunday morning. He expected her to be dressed, in her wheelchair and ready to roll. He took her across town to Sunday services at her old home church.

His mother, Alice, was quite debilitated with arthritis and osteoporosis. Getting her dressed to her satisfaction was one of our most time consuming efforts and came with his very specific time frame - every Sunday. Mother was always ready, meticulously groomed and dressed to the nines. She was forever pleasant and smiling when her son appeared at 9:00 a.m., no matter how short the Sunday staffing, no matter how many resident problems or emergencies had surfaced that morning.

The nursing staff also knew her son would deliver a fresh baked pie every Sunday morning. The only question was what kind of pie today?

Alice was forever pleasant, but oblivious to the demands her Sunday schedule placed on the entire staff. She was confined to a large motorized wheelchair necessitated by her size. She could barely manage the controls with her deformed fingers that protruded from her wrist and hand braces. Additional splints and supports for her neck, elbows, knees, ankles and feet needed to be affixed perfectly over her sensitive skin. Each device had to be applied slowly and then wait for Alice's approval before moving to the next. Finally, numerous pillows were tucked around her body for comfort.

On Sunday mornings she had her alarm set for 6:00 a.m. Her routine required two nurse's aides (CNAs) to transfer her into the wheelchair, take her to the bathroom, lift her onto the toilet and subsequently off the toilet.

Alice was in the dining room before 7:00 a.m. where the kitchen staff had prepared her breakfast tray early. A nursing assistant very patiently spoon-fed Alice who seemed to chew and swallow in slow motion. The process was slowed by Alice's casual never-ending conversation, which could not be ignored, because she asked questions and expected answers.

When finally returned to her room the slow task of selecting her attire for the day began. Her vintage wardrobe was beautifully adorned with buttons, ribbons, lace, ruffles and delicate stitching and all posed problems during the dressing process. Most of her joints were frozen and allowed no flexibility when donning the frills.

After her clothing was laid out two nurse's aides were needed to lift her onto the shower chair. She preferred Maria to help with her showers because Maria knew her preferences, such as how hard to scrub her back and when to turn the water on or off. Shower complete, clock ticking, Maria wrapped Alice and the shower chair in a sheet, leaving nothing but her head visible. She rolled the package to the full-length mirror beside the bed and began to blow-dry Alice's hair while the pleasant conversation and questions continued.

A second nurse's aide was required to move her back into her wheelchair and then stand her long enough to slip her dress and petticoat over her head and stiff arms then down over her body. Alice thought nylon stockings were necessary although braces covered them. Shoes were especially hard to fit over her gnarled feet. She watched in the mirror while Maria slipped on her necklace, earrings and intricate hair clips.

She insisted on trying to do everything for herself but could do very little. Maria allowed her to attempt each individual grooming chore, always in slow motion, always methodical, always with more time lost due to her chitchat. After all the delay she allowed Maria to complete the task and they moved on the next one with the same sequence.

Finally, Alice directed as Maria wrapped a shawl and lap robe around her body. They had mastered concealing the braces, but left her stunning dress and accessories visible.

Her son appeared at 9:00 a.m., tall, handsome, svelte, tailored dark suit, matching coal black hair sported a trendy masculine trim and polished shoes reflected the ceiling light's brightness. His starched white shirt, gold cufflinks and gray silk tie were mere accents to his manly features and exquisite taste.

"Good morning, Angela." He handed the nurse a pie.

His gaze and attention quickly turned to his mother motoring toward him. "Well, good morning Mrs. Johnson, aren't you beautiful today. I'm so glad you wore that yellow dress, you'll brighten up the entire service." He nodded discreet approval to staff, while continuing the lighthearted conversation with Alice. He lost no time opening the door with a gentleman's gesture and Alice motored tenuously over the threshold.

I watched from the window; his gentle, efficient lift moved Alice from the wheelchair to the car seat, then he loaded the heavy electric chair onto the rear ramp and sped away. Alice's elegance was visible from the passenger window.

By now the all-female staff was enjoying pecan pie with vanilla ice cream confiscated from the kitchen. Their discussion of Mr. Johnson was spirited. Over time they pieced together enough information to understand his devotion to Alice. He cared for her at home over many years and told one of them, "I do not have time for a marriage and family as long as Mother's alive."

A middle-aged nursing assistant summed up their collective gossip, "What a shameful waste of a good man."

This example illustrates the success of an advocate's clear, consistent request. Although difficult for the staff they respected his devotion and understood their work for the day would be far more pleasant if they fulfilled his request. The pie was a small token, but it warranted a break in the morning routine. Yet, his nodded approval was far more important.

EXAMPLE: Gifting as advocacy.

Changes in management and deteriorating care in Mother's first nursing home demanded that I find better care. I chose the facility closest to my home because it seemed all the area facilities presented similar obstacles like poor staffing and disorder during my visits. I called a nurse friend with years of work experience in surrounding nursing homes. She lent her endorsement, "Frances, it's no worse than any of the others around here."

I used the plan listed above and set about finding a couple of good nurses and nurse's aides early in her admission. I was looking for honest, attentive, smart nurses and nurse's aides with tenure. I thought I might need their future help since Mother was pretty healthy and spry for eighty-nine years, just very confused most of the time.

An early hassle with Mother was her preoccupation with a shower before bed. We were discouraged from pursuing that objective because there was not enough staff for evening showers, it did not fit the nursing home's routine and other dismal reasons why it was not possible. Long after the shower issue had been forgotten I handed a kind, caring, nurse's aide a plain Easter card with no name, no signature and a $20 bill inside. No one saw me make the pass and I did not tell Mother. She was soon receiving showers in the evening and told me about getting her nails trimmed and a few other niceties.

I appreciated a helpful, considerate nurse who worked the evening shift and thanked him with a birthday card and enclosed $50 bill. I greeted him with "Happy Birthday Ray," placed the card on his medicine cart where he was working and left the building. There was no one else in the hall and no name or signature on the card. Again, Mother was not aware and Ray never mentioned it. However, his personal involvement heightened with added attention toward getting Mother to bed every night: Directing a nurse's aide to find a nightgown, reassurance that all her stuff was safe, "I'm taking care of it Mrs. Vance, everything's okay," then her anti-anxiety medication to assure a good night's sleep.

Important to this type of advocacy was my selectivity and the integrity of the employees. Without any identification the employee could not be targeted if discovered. They could be fired for accepting anything from a resident, but I thought I could claim innocence— just giving a gift—if the employee reported me to administration. No problems arose and there were additional occasions. I always presented the gifts in association with holidays, birthdays and anniversaries.

A reminder to readers: This guide is written for the purpose of helping to navigate nursing home systems - it is not an ethics manifesto. If you have problems with this type of advocacy, don't do it.

EXAMPLE: One daughter's solution to overseeing her mother's care from a distance.

I first learned of gifting possibilities from my cousin June. She cried uncontrollably as she described her mother's circumstances. Nursing home placement of her parents near their home and friends worked well until her father passed away. They shared a room and he supervised Mother's care, but in his absence she deteriorated. She was weak and frail, but alert. Arthritic deformities of her hands left her unable to feed herself. The nursing home reported a serious weight loss.

June lived in a distant city. On an unannounced visit she found her mother's lunch tray sitting in front of her, untouched and cold. Family members reported similar observations on their visits. Her report to the charge nurse proved noncommittal and disappointing.

She returned the next day to find a young nurse's aide, Sally, feeding her mother. Over the next few days she noticed that when Sally was Mother's assigned nurse's aide (CNA) she was fed, bathed, positioned and turned with care.

June was distressed. She decided to give Sally $20 cash and ask for help . . . "Just make sure Mother gets fed when I'm not here." The arrangement worked well and grew. Gifts continued. June knew her mother was fed. Sally watched over her care and discreetly called after leaving work when problems developed.

My cousin's reasoning and justification are noteworthy. "Those poor aides get paid slave wages, their benefits are a farce and they get treated like s _ _ _! Sally can use that extra money for her kids." She insisted the cash paid to Sally was nothing more than a "thank you" and a gift.

References

OMBUDSMAN: An advocate (supporter) who works to solve problems between residents and their nursing homes and assisted living facilities. Ombudsmen have no designated authority but carry considerable clout within facilities. Websites for state programs are usually located within each state's office on aging. https://www.medicare.gov/claims-and-appeals/medicare-rights/get-help/ombudsman.html

Consumer Voice Clearinghouse: National Consumer Voice for Quality Long-Term Care: 1) Information for LTC consumers, including fact sheets regarding individualized care (individuals living in nursing homes, assisted living, or receiving home and community-based care) http://theconsumervoice.org/issues/recipients

ADVOCACY

2) Resources for family members
http://theconsumervoice.org/issues/family
3) Resources for advocates (resident-directed care information and fact sheets) http://theconsumervoice.org/issues/for-advocates

Kaiser Health News: "Volunteers Help Ombudsmen Give Nursing Home Residents 'A Voice' In Their Care," by Susan Jaffe, May 2, 2017

The New York Times: "Poor Patient Care at Many Nursing Homes Despite Stricter Oversight," by Jordan Rau, July 5, 2017. https://nyti.ms/2tOdkOp

ABUSE: The OIG (Office of Inspector General) preliminary report: Early Alert: The Centers for Medicare & Medicaid Services Has Inadequate Procedures To Ensure That Incidents of Potential Abuse or Neglect at Skilled Nursing Facilities Are Identified and Reported in Accordance With Applicable Requirements, page 1, A-01-17-00504 (Aug. 24, 2017), at https://oig.hhs.gov/oas/reports/region1/11700504.pdf

CHAPTER 22

THE CAREGIVERS

A nursing home book would not be complete without a look at the caregivers--nurses and nurses' aides. Every nursing home resident needs assistance with some daily activity (hygiene, bathing, dressing, eating, toileting) and nursing staff provides that personal care. Additionally, they give emotional support, a safe environment and medications around the clock. Thus, the term caregivers.

I often hear sympathy for "the work they do" referencing the cleanup of urine and feces, bathing, dressing and feeding messy, confused residents. This refrain is often followed by, "and they don't get paid anything." All nursing personnel have completed licensing and certification programs providing exposure and experience in the chores often shunned by others. Each understands and accepts the nature of their duties. Cleanups are burdensome only when inadequate numbers of staff and supplies limit the time and attention essential to assisting an incontinent or untidy resident.

Most caretakers proudly defend the time spent on menial personal tasks as an essential part of their job. Such attention is a source of comfort and self-esteem for residents and pride for caregivers. You need see only one beaming nurse's aide and thankful resident, clean-shaven, sharply dressed in his khaki pants, white shirt and polished shoes to understand their incentive. A "thank you" from the resident or family adds to the day's pleasure. The time carved from a busy schedule to meticulously braid a bright ribbon into a comatose resident's hair is a source of pride for the nurse's aide and adds cheer to everyone's day. I am inclined to believe that even a comatose resident is aware of such tenderness.

Training programs do not prepare nurses and nurses' aides for the volume of work most facilities expect of them. Weariness often sets in when limited time, help and supplies deny them the opportunity to do a good job. Poor resident care weighs heavily on the conscience of dedicated caregivers. They are further demoralized when concerns of resident care and safety are ignored and often considered a complaint. Newcomers to nursing home employment soon learn that caregivers with complaints about resident care are disposable.

Caregivers in many facilities face degradation of their personal and professional worth. Their skill, expertise and insight have little or no value to corporate ownership. Appreciation for their dedication in spite of daily hurdles is absent. Threats of replacing them if they can't complete their assignments are often the norm. The impossible task of providing good care is a leading reason for burnout.

In the past working as a nurses' aide was a career choice for many women. The job offered opportunities for a sustainable livelihood with performance raises, a few benefits and employment stability. With the advent of venture capital and corporate interests, nursing home employment has become transient and volatile for both nurses' aides and nurses. Frequent changes in management and ownership guarantee employment and financial insecurity. I have seen the enthusiasm of many new caregivers wane under the stress of their job's uncertainty.

In the midst of turmoil, a few nursing homes operate outside the corporate model. Independent owners of facilities are more likely to nurture caregivers, thus providing a degree of stability for both staff and residents.

The BE AWARE and BEWARE sections provide insight into the molding of caregiver attitudes. The EXAMPLES are an attempt to show how caregiver attitudes weave their way into resident care.

BE AWARE
- Physical characteristics, race or gender are not predictors of any caregiver's value. I am accustomed to the most unlikely showing the greatest sensitivity and devotion to their residents. Among them were burly, tattooed men, former truck drivers, probable gang members and Katrina evacuees desperate for work while suffering their own despair.
- The worth of nurse's aides goes far beyond physical care. They spend more time with residents than any other staff members and have intimate knowledge of their needs. Their observations are invaluable.
- Nurse's aide pay often begins at minimum wage with a national average of $10 per hour. Opportunities for raises are rare.

Changes in ownership mean each employee starts off as a new-hire of the new company at base wage.
- Too often, careers are harmed by vindictive employers listing an employee as "not eligible for rehire." This reality often leads to voluntary resignations because this branding signals "troublemaker" to any other employer calling for a work reference.
- When issues of resident care arise nurses are often blamed for errors and accidents even when they have no control over short staffing, limited supplies and faulty equipment. Corporations have finessed the art of threatening to report a nurse in such circumstances to the State Nursing Board as incompetent. Now the nurse faces the possibility of losing their professional license and career. Subsequently, the nurse is given the option of resigning voluntarily to avoid the report and they have little choice but to do so. The benefit to corporate owners is a shift of responsibility to the nurse (evidenced by the resignation) which dampens the possibility of legal action and calms a responsible party because this "bad nurse" is gone and will no longer be taking care of their loved one.
- The prevailing attitude of corporate ownership is that every caregiver can be replaced. No thought is given to how staff changes impact resident care and wellbeing. Therefore, caregiver's employment longevity becomes important when comparing nursing homes.
- Nursing home caregivers migrate from one employment setting to another. The norm is to continue friendships and contacts with peers. In so doing, networks develop keeping nurses and nurses' aides up to date on the status of care in the area's competitors. Sometimes objectivity is lost when looking at their current employment. At other times they see their nursing home's shortcomings, but manage adversity by doing the best they can and hoping for future improvement.
- Most nurses and nurse's aides look at employment on a day-to-day basis. They tolerate adverse circumstances as long as they feel they took good care of their assigned residents at shift's end. Ultimately, most caregivers accept and work within the status quo.

- National Bureau of Labor statistics show nurse's aides are second only to loading dock laborers in sustaining on-the-job injuries. Most are back injuries which trigger an immediate offensive from management to fault the employee (did not follow lifting protocol, did not wait for lifting help, did not use a mechanical lift, etc.). The injured are at a greater disadvantage when the employer has opted out of the state workers compensation insurance and set up their own self-insured program for injured workers.
- Personal difficulties outside the facility may impact a caregiver's performance. As an example, a caregiver seems distant while feeding a resident. She offers no conversation or interaction. Could the stress of a flat tire on the way to work, no spare tire, a reprimand for being late, no transportation to pick up a baby at daycare and children after school, no money to fix the flat or buy a tire have a single mother totally preoccupied because she is afoot with payday a week away?

BEWARE
- The approach nurses and nurses' aides use in caring for their residents reflects their individual personalities. Seek out those showing kindness, respect, humor, gentleness, patience, engaging in conversation and admiration of residents.
- The majority will do their best to complete their daily assignments with the least possible stress from supervisors, residents or visitors. On the fringes are the very bad and very good. It is worthwhile to ferret out the very good and cultivate a trusting relationship with each.
- Caregiver duties are quite structured. Nurses take care of medications, treatments, doctor's orders, schedules and emergencies. Nurse's aides take care of residents—hygiene, dressing, toileting, feeding, exercise and conversation. Suggestions are better targeted at the right caregiver and requests are usually far more productive than complaints.
- Be prepared for your caregiver connections to be severed by the uncertainties of nursing home employment, e.g., resignations, terminations and ownership changes. As your task of identifying the very good begins anew you will gain a healthy

respect for those nursing homes providing employment stability and longevity.
- Caregiver abuse, including texting of compromising resident photos, is cause for alarm; yet the industry shuns accountability. In most instances the employee is terminated for a minor and unrelated cause and moves on to another facility.

EXAMPLE: Every caregiver recalls a few unforgettable residents. Ms. Dora was one of those because she always seemed to have the upper hand with staff.

Ms. Dora came to the nursing home several weeks earlier for treatment for a huge pressure sore on her lower back and pelvic area. She was a rail thin, tall, black lady with penetrating eyes and prominent arthritic joints. By now she was familiar with the routine of positioning, cleaning and treating her wound.

Nurses dreaded the process because the wound was deep and care complicated. Ms. Dora's unpredictable responses created additional stress. She was always a loose cannon. She might start screaming, cursing, and fighting at any time during the process. She often screamed at the top of her lungs, "POLICE, POLICE. Help, Help, They're molesting me." She had screeched, "Sluts. Bitches. Whores."

I walked into her room on a Sunday morning to explain that it was time to take care of her "sore." The head of her bed was rolled up, she sipped coffee in comfort at 10 am. She had a different program on her TV, not the usual Sunday morning church services or novelas the staff turns TVs to while working in rooms.

"Good morning, Ms. Dora. How are you today?"

"I'm fine."

"What are you watching?"

"Face the Nation."

"Well, who is that guy?" I asked.

"Bob Scheiffer! Youuuu . . .doooon't . . . eeeeven . . . knooow . . . whooooo . . . Boooob . . . Scheeeeifer . . . is!"

"Well I do now, Ms. Dora. Thank you for teaching me something." We watched until the next commercial. Then I asked, "Can we take care of your sore?"

"If I can watch 'Face the Nation' while you do it."

I summoned her nurse, "Hurry, before we lose Bob Scheiffer."

It became the easiest wound care ever, not even a whimper from Ms. Dora. Her attention and eyes stayed glued to "Face the Nation."

EXAMPLE: Nurses and nurse's aides often face heart-wrenching situations, which are difficult to understand. As they search for answers, their only consolation is mutual love and the opportunity to make the resident's journey easier. Willie was such a resident.

The usually delightful charge nurse, Anita, approached me in a forlorn mood. "Frances, please help me with Willie. You know I do his wound care last because it hurts me and it hurts him so bad. The odor's been really awful the last few days."

I worked weekends so I hadn't seen Willie's wounds for a week, but I knew him well: quiet, gentle, considerate, respectful in spite of his painful terminal cancer. His wife was equally memorable. She sat quietly at his bedside, all day long every day. She hadn't arrived yet, most likely at church. I pictured her and Willie as the quintessential Southeast San Antonio family.

After giving Willie strong pain medication and waiting for it to take effect, three of us gathered around the treatment cart parked outside Willie's door. Anita took her own sweet time to collect and prepare supplies. She explained to me that his nurse's aide, Lupe, would be helping us today. "She wants to go to nursing school. I told her, 'Then you need to come help with Willie. This will show you what nursing's really like.'"

We took a final inventory of supplies before entering the room. Any delay to retrieve missed articles would prolong Willie's pain. Anita and I nodded agreement; we had everything we needed. Lupe watched anxiously.

We slipped into the room. Each moved in slow motion to take a pair of gloves from the box on the wall. We tried to be quiet. No need to awaken Willie a minute too soon. He seemed so cozy and comfortable. Only his small, gaunt, coal black face was visible in a cloud of white sheets. Anita maneuvered around the foot of the bed, determined not to bump the bed or furniture in the crowded room.

Anita is a contradiction—middle-aged, overweight, frazzled, ringlets of strawberry blond hair adorn her forehead, yet she is reminiscent of a ballerina. She balances her dressings at shoulder level in one hand, her bandage scissors held high in the other but never taking mournful eyes off her peaceful patient. She positioned herself at the bedside and gingerly placed her dressings on a clean area of the bedside table. She stood at the bedside for several minutes just looking at Willie while Lupe and I stood in reverence.

Willie had wrapped himself tightly in his sheet with only his face visible. Nonetheless, the tight contours of the sheet outlined his emaciated body with little more than skin and bone remaining of his small frame.

"Papa, I love you," Anita said, barely above a whisper.

"I love you baby," Willie replied as he opened his weary eyes and looked into hers. He did not move another muscle.

"You know I love you, Papa," Lupe said, then placed her soft hand on his shoulder.

"I know baby, I know," Willie replied, barely audible.

With mutual love and understanding the grim and painful task of removing old, soaked bandages began in silence. The gangrenous smell was nauseating and almost overwhelming, but none of us hinted we were working in anything other than his own rose garden. Lupe didn't flinch. Her jaw was set and hands were steady as she peered at the extensive sores all around his foot. The left leg Lupe and I held suspended in the air became heavier and heavier as Anita gently cleansed the exposed tendon and bone. The wounds were extensive and worsening.

After finishing, we rested Willie's foot back on the bed, then the three of us stood up straight, rested for about a minute and took a deep breath. We needed relief for our strained back muscles. Now we could begin the right foot, we knew it to be just as demanding for us and painful for Willie.

Anita broke the long silence. "Papa, I'm gonna take care of your other foot now."

"Okay baby, okay." He tightened his grip on the bedrails.

Lupe and I strained to suspend and position his right leg so Anita could see the wound. She worked with precision through the treatment. A reassuring touch on Willie's forehead or shoulder would have comforted him, but all six hands were engaged in our primary task.

As we finished and repositioned Willie to his preferred right side he gripped the bedrails with both hands. I tried to reassure him we were finished, he could turn loose the rails and try to relax.

"I'm okay, ma'am, I'm okay." His voice trembled; his eyes closed as if he wished to escape his surroundings.

I rearranged the pillow in a final attempt to provide comfort. His arthritic hands did not move from the bedrails, but seemed to strain for a tighter grip. Lupe and I gathered the trash before leaving. Anita took a last look at Willie and shook her head—she had nothing more to offer.

We were relieved to find his wife waiting in the hall; he would be okay now. She was not flustered to learn that Willie's wounds were worse, just glad his ordeal was over for the day. Lupe listened intently as we talked with Willie's wife then disappeared down the hallway to care for other residents.

Anita and I were exhausted. We sat at the nurse's station trying to regain our strength. I asked, "So, is Lupe nurse material?"

"Yep, she can take care of me any day."

CHAPTER 23

EPILOGUE

During the 2009 healthcare debate, fears of "pulling the plug on granny" and "death panels" became the protective stance of a few politicians. Nine years later these pseudo sympathizers have done nothing to intervene in the "plug pulling" which occurs every single day in multiple nursing homes across the country. The reality is that "pulling the plug" is not a humane separation from a power source as the term implies. Such an event would probably result in a reasonably painless, quick death.

Under current conditions pulling the plug in a nursing home is usually a slow, downward spiral of preventable events. The result is less than humane and never quick. Consider the resident who does not receive help eating, becomes malnourished, weak, bedridden, develops bedsores which become infected, causing dehydration and death.

Politicians rail sanctimoniously about their concern for nursing home residents. Nursing homes' corporate owners and lobbyists whine to the same politicians about needing more Medicare and Medicaid reimbursement while the plight of nursing home patients remains largely forgotten.

Nursing home trade groups promote their industry as the most regulated in the country, but fail to reveal their success in fighting enforcement of these same regulations. Individual complaints and media investigations repeatedly encounter the impotence of state regulatory agencies. Nursing home employees understand the coziness of many *state* inspectors to the ownership. They also see the frustration and turnover of those inspectors attempting objective inspections.

On the other hand, *federal* inspectors from the U.S. Department of Health and Human Services (USDHHS) entering the front door alarms ownership. They always arrive unannounced and unexpected. USDHHS (the *feds*, as referred to by the industry) inspectors are serious and detached from local and state political influence. Their observations and audits can result in cut-off of federal funds, or even worse, recoup money already paid. However, there are few federal inspections.

The Affordable Care Act attempts to fight top-level nursing home fraud, improve transparency and raise ethics standards. The Center for Medicare and Medicaid Services (CMS) issued new patient centered regulations in late 2016. The three-year phase-in began in 2017, but the guidelines have been reversed for 2018. Additionally, fines against nursing homes that harm residents or place them at grave risk of injury have been scaled back. The impact on residents' lives is predictable.

Some feel their only personal option is to avoid nursing home admission. Alternative plans are often dashed when sobering reality reveals that nursing home care has become necessary. When the nursing home experience ends, those impacted by poor care tend to move on, relieved that their loved one's trauma is behind them.

On a larger scale, citizens care about the fate of nursing home residents. They express outrage when media exposes nursing home abuse and neglect. Claims by the industry or their trade organizations that these conditions and circumstances are isolated remain unfounded. They have been successful in hiding the numbers with arbitration clauses and settlements shielded from public records and scrutiny.

CMS's capitulation on the 2018 guidelines which centered on patient care underscores ownership and management's long-standing ability to divert attention from substandard care to their mantra-lack of resources. An example: the industry remains successful in killing any legislation setting nurse-to-resident staffing ratios even though overwhelming evidence proves that increasing nursing hours improves resident care.

Administrators and professionals within each building determine their own approach, but shortcomings are still explained with the familiar excuse - not enough federal reimbursement to provide the care residents need. This explanation has worked for the majority of nursing homes for years and it remains effective today. There are exceptions. A limited number of facilities provide good care with the same reimbursement amounts as their competitors who are delivering the worst of care.

Nursing home employees tend to look at care from their immediate working situation rather than industry-wide issues. Most accept barriers to care as the norm, yet feel that they take good care of their own residents in spite of hindrances. I recall one administrator who complained about the care her mother was receiving in a different nursing home, but could not see the same problems in our facility.

For those employees who recognize the extent of problems, there are insurmountable obstacles to being heard. Nurses can claim *safe harbor* (similar to whistleblower protections) in a few states, but this route is most often a dead end of administrative hurdles and a lost career. Caregivers' only option is to move from one facility to another following promises of better working conditions, the opportunity to do a good job and sometimes higher pay.

Are there answers? Yes! However, any solutions will come from outside the industry. I encourage attention to nursing home issues when they arise, both locally and nationally. Why? The public's investment is vast. Consider the private dollars (pensions, social security checks and resource spenddowns) which go toward care. Then there are the tax dollars funneled through Medicare and Medicaid.

A starting point is transparency. Politicians will be more interested in following tax money when constituents are asking questions. What percentage is spent on resident care and what percentage goes toward administrative fees and bonuses? How much is spent on lobbying and campaign contributions? If public interest was strong, how long would it take policymakers to remove forced arbitration clauses from admission contracts, thus restoring residents' right to a jury trial?

The need for nursing home care has never been greater and the number needing the care is increasing. Anyone who has struggled through the taxing duties of twenty-four-hour care acknowledges the relief obtained with their loved one's nursing home admission. Many of us will become that loved one who needs care. The price paid for care seems insignificant when resources are available and the need is great. Cost becomes an issue in the presence of substandard care. Facilities which fulfill the promise of good care and remain profitable stand out as models.

The rapid pace of investment and expansions indicate nursing homes remain a profitable endeavor. Few consumers question the necessity of profits, but the question of profit *margins* arises when guidelines for improving resident care are delayed by outcries of needing more money. Total transparency could justify the need for increased reimbursement. In the meantime, we still have the model of the few profitable nursing homes taking good care of their residents.

APPENDIX A: Star Ratings

The CMS Five-Star Rating System

The star rating system is a merging of official statistics and facility reported information. Star ratings tackle four areas: inspections, staffing, quality measures and overall ratings. Inspections are conducted by state agencies and become official statistics. Staffing and quality measures have historically been reported by the nursing homes and therefore considered self-reported. The scope of the overall star is limited to a complex formula of information based on inspections, staffing and quality measures.

The Five-Star Rating System was initiated in 2008 with reviews and updates ongoing since its beginning. The staff rating was added in 2013 after CMS acknowledged that resident care is usually better when more staff is available. Antianxiety/hypnotic medications were added and then removed from the quality measures.

Resident advocates have consistently directed attention to shortcomings, especially in the self-reported areas. During 2016 some of their suggestions were realized in improved data collection for staffing and a few of the quality measures. Additionally, by looking at short-stay residents you are now able to compare facilities' rehabilitation statistics.

Short-stay residents, those in-building 100 days or less, are generally Medicare clients admitted for therapy and skilled care. You can compare facility percentages for how many recovered and returned home, had to return to the hospital or emergency room, or remained in the nursing home.

Overall Rating

The overall star rating is a composite of the three individual star ratings: inspections, staffing and quality measures. The core of the overall rating is the health inspection rating, which is adjusted up if the facility receives very high staffing or quality measure ratings, and is adjusted down for low staffing or quality measure ratings.

The *overall* rating is not a reflection of the whole facility but a merging of data already presented in the other star categories: inspections, staffing and quality measures.

APPENDIX A

Inspections

Annual inspections involve two aspects, safety and health. The safety inspection refers to the building's safety: fire alarms, sprinkler systems, emergency power, building codes, etc. Sometimes referred to as the Life Safety Code, none of these findings are included in the Five-Star Rating System.

The inspection referred to in the five-star rating is the health inspection. It is based on the last three annual inspections plus any complaint investigations during that time. Although there are eighteen components of the health inspection, the five-star ratings only consider eleven.

CMS five-star inspection ratings are based on the relative performance of facilities within a state rather than a national comparison. Therefore, expect variations when comparing facilities in different states.

Facility inspection ratings are determined by using a method similar to the Bell Curve: The best 10 percent in each state receive a five-star rating; the middle 70 percent receive a rating of two, three, or four stars, with approximately 23.33 percent in each rating category; the worst 20 percent receive a one-star rating.

- CMS contracts with the state regulatory agencies to conduct health and safety inspections, complaint investigations and certifications that new facilities meet minimum standards. Timeliness of reporting this information varies by state, but once posted, the *inspection date* is important. It may be several months old.
- Federal inspectors check on the state inspectors' work to make sure they are following the national process and differences between states stay within reasonable bounds. Federal inspections are rare.
- Information gathered at the state level is transmitted to CMS and becomes the inspection component of star rating calculations. The timeliness and content of inspections varies by state. Therefore, the CMS website may not reflect the results of the last inspection completed.
- In most instances these statistics will have been compiled when a facility is providing its best care during a few days of the inspection and do not reflect baseline operation during the remainder of the year.

- Although inspections are unscheduled and unannounced each facility expects an inspection within a few weeks before or after the last annual inspection date, referred to as their "window."
- Intense preparation to update documentation, staffing and patient care is the norm during this window and continues until the inspection is complete.
- Rarely will the staffing ratios and level of care provided during an inspection be maintained after inspectors leave the building.
- Corporate owners routinely send in "swat teams" to prepare for inspections and help clear known problems. The goal is not to provide long-term solutions and improved care but to avoid deficiencies and fines imposed during the inspection.
- If an inspection team finds that a nursing home doesn't meet a minimum standard in a specific area it issues a deficiency citation. Both the state and federal agencies may assess a fine, deny payment to the nursing home, assign a temporary manager, or install a state monitor. Penalties are determined by the severity and extent of deficiencies.

Nursing homes are notorious for calling in extra staff during inspections thus tainting information collected by the inspectors. The additional staff improves chances for fewer deficiencies and a good inspection report. Also evident is how the same level of staffing would improve residents' daily care when inspectors are not in the building.

- With added nursing assistants available to provide personal attention, deficiencies in key areas of inspector attention can be avoided:
    1. Staff appears less rushed and more attentive to residents.
    2. All residents are well groomed.
    3. Incontinent episodes are attended to immediately.
    4. Residents are fed on time and provided all the help needed during meals.
    5. Call bells and lights are answered promptly.
    6. Noisy call bell systems will not be muted.
    7. Inspectors hear fewer complaints from residents and families.
- More nurses on duty decreases the risk of unwanted attention in focus areas where one error can trigger intense scrutiny and

probable deficiencies. Additionally, nurses are better able to supervise and oversee care:
1. Medications, treatments and feedings are provided on time.
2. The possibility of errors decreases.
3. More housekeepers avoid environmental attention of inspectors.
4. Rooms are clean; hallway floors are spotless and shining.
5. Trash and dirty linen are removed promptly; odors receive immediate attention.
6. Housekeepers have time to follow infection control measures for their equipment such as mops, brooms and gloves.

For years facilities have used hospital admissions to cover up bad care and avoid deficiencies. When nursing home management knows they will be cited for especially bad care on individual residents they send them to the hospital when inspectors arrive. Questions about their care will not arise during inspection because both the residents and their medical records are out of sight.

The recent transition to collecting data on short-stay residents' transfers to the hospital and emergency room may be helpful in identifying these practices. Results remain to be seen. Long stay residents, those in the nursing home over 100 days, and Medicare Advantage clients are not included in this tracking.

Staffing

In 2013 CMS recognized the significant impact of staffing on resident care and added a star category for those statistics. Many facilities dropped one or two stars as a result. The rating for staffing is adjusted for different levels of resident care. That is, nursing homes with residents who need more care versus residents needing less attention.

- A few states have staffing standards, but the nursing home industry has been able to block federal requirements for staffing hours.
- The staffing hours are an average spread across the total number of residents not an allotment for each patient.
- Staffing data were previously self-reported only once a year and were collected two weeks prior to an inspection. Staffing has

probably been better during this period as the facility readies for an inspection. By the end of 2016 CMS implemented a quarterly electronic reporting system that is auditable back to facility payrolls in order to verify staffing information.
- Advocates and CMS both note that quality is generally better in nursing homes that have more staff working directly with residents.

Quality Measures

The standard form, the Minimum Data Set (MDS), is used to collect resident care information and ultimately determines quality measures. Each resident's data are collected at three-month intervals, beginning on their admission date, then reported to CMS who updates monthly. The quality measures are gathered and self-reported by the facility.

This information is not audited by CMS so it must be interpreted cautiously. The possibility of inaccurate information entering into the quality measures is a shortcoming, which leaves facilities reporting accurately at a disadvantage.
- When facing submission deadlines or in the case of a lazy employee there is a temptation to click through the program's checklist with little attention to residents' conditions. Thus inaccurate information is entered into the quality measures.
- Residents' improvement or deterioration is determined by comparing the last three reports from each resident.
- Most of the quality measures reflect residents' conditions during the 7 days before the assessment was done. Therefore, the quality measures may not represent the residents' clinical conditions during the entire time period between assessments.
- Short staffing and administrative pressure often force the most conscientious employees to choose between patient care and using their precious time for charting. Perhaps a resident's shower must wait until tomorrow, because it must be charted on time—that is, today—even though it was not done today.
- In most facilities, one registered nurse is responsible for quality measures data entry and is called the MDS coordinator. Experienced MDS coordinators—expert at understanding the program pathways and meeting deadlines—are among the highest paid employees in the building.

APPENDIX A

All data collection places great emphasis on whether a condition such as malnutrition, dehydration, infections, bedsores etc. developed in the nursing home (in-house, facility acquired, nosocomial) or whether the resident had the condition when they arrived at the nursing home (community or hospital acquired).
- Often in-house conditions such as bedsores and malnutrition are never documented in the medical record, therefore they never appear in the nursing home statistics.
- Under-reporting of in-house conditions abounds and thus distorts a major problem to seem less significant when it appears in nursing home reports and statistics.
  1. Severe deep bedsores are often documented as shallow skin ulcers, abrasions and blisters.
  2. Malnutrition and dehydration may simply appear as weight loss on documentation because the facility does not want to obtain needed lab work. To do so would identify the gravity of the resident's condition. Once identified the malnourished resident requires additional resources within the nursing home: a treatment plan, supplements, consultations and additional staff attention.
  3. Many falls are never recorded in residents' records therefore they are never captured in the nursing home statistics.
- Hospital admissions are used to cover up bad statistics.
  1. Even though an in-house condition such as an infection requires hospital admission it is reclassified as hospital acquired on return to the nursing home. The nursing home has then cleared the record of an undesirable in-house statistic.
  2. If a resident is hospitalized for two or three days a new admission record is usually begun when the resident returns to the facility. The old chart is closed giving the nursing home a new start. Even though the resident's bedsore, malnutrition, dehydration, broken hip and pneumonia were all present when they left the nursing home, the new record shows a new admission arriving with the conditions—now hospital or community

acquired. The nursing home has deflected their own responsibility to the hospital.
3. The resident's old record is closed and the undesirable statistics are buried in medical records as a discharged resident. Rarely will an inspector ask for a closed chart.
- The Affordable Care Act (ACA) initiated new rules to track nursing home and hospital admissions and readmissions. So far, there is no data on hospital admissions associated with inspection dates.
- It remains to be seen whether the move to electronic records will improve transparency and the quality of data collection.
- The technical manual found on the CMS website offers additional information on the Five-Star Rating System.

APPENDIX B: Resident's Rights

What are my rights in a nursing home?
As a nursing home resident, you have certain rights and protections under Federal and state law that help ensure you get the care and services you need. You have the right to be informed, make your own decisions, and have your personal information kept private.

The nursing home must tell you about these rights and explain them in writing in a language you understand. They must also explain in writing how you should act and what you're responsible for while you're in the nursing home. This must be done before or at the time you're admitted, as well as during your stay. You must acknowledge in writing that you got this information.

At a minimum, Federal law specifies that nursing homes must protect and promote the following rights of each resident. You have the right to:
- **Be Treated with Respect:** You have the right to be treated with dignity and respect, as well as make your own schedule and participate in the activities you choose. You have the right to decide when you go to bed, rise in the morning, and eat your meals.
- **Participate in Activities:** You have the right to participate in an activities program designed to meet your needs and the needs of the other residents.
- **Be Free from Discrimination:** Nursing homes don't have to accept all applicants, but they must comply with Civil Rights laws that say they can't discriminate based on race, color, national origin, disability, age, or religion. The Department of Health and Human Services, Office for Civil Rights has more information. Visit http://www.hhs.gov/ocr.
- **Be Free from Abuse and Neglect:** You have the right to be free from verbal, sexual, physical, and mental abuse. Nursing homes can't keep you apart from everyone else against your will. If you feel you have been mistreated (abused) or the nursing home isn't meeting your needs (neglect), report this to the nursing home, your family, your local Long-Term Care

Ombudsman, or State Survey Agency. The nursing home must investigate and report all suspected violations and any injuries of unknown origin within 5 working days of the incident to the proper authorities.
- **Be Free from Restraints:** Nursing homes can't use any physical restraints (like side rails) or chemical restraints (like drugs) to discipline you for the staff's own convenience.
- **Make Complaints:** You have the right to make a complaint to the staff of the nursing home, or any other person, without fear of punishment. The nursing home must address the issue promptly.

Get Proper Medical Care: You have the following rights regarding your medical care:
- To be fully informed about your total health status in a language you understand.
- To be fully informed about your medical condition, prescription and over-the-counter drugs, vitamins, and supplements.
- To be involved in the choice of your doctor.
- To participate in the decisions that affects your care.
- To take part in developing your care plan. By law, nursing homes must develop a care plan for each resident. You have the right to take part in this process. Family members can also help with your care plan with your permission.
- To access all your records and reports, including clinical records (medical records and reports) promptly (on weekdays). Your legal guardian has the right to look at all your medical records and make important decisions on your behalf.
- To express any complaints (sometimes called "grievances") you have about your care or treatment.
- To create advance directives (a health care proxy or power of attorney, a living will, after-death wishes) in accordance with State law.
- To refuse to participate in experimental treatment.

Have Your Representative Notified: The nursing home must notify your doctor and, if known, your legal representative or an interested family member when the following occurs:

- You're involved in an accident and are injured and/or need to see a doctor.
- Your physical, mental, or psychosocial status starts to get worse.
- You have a life threatening condition.
- You have medical complications.
- Your treatment needs to change significantly.
- The nursing home decides to transfer or discharge you from the nursing home.

Get Information on Services and Fees: You have the right to be told in writing about all nursing home services and fees (those that are charged and not charged to you) before you move into the nursing home and at any time when services and fees change. In addition:
- The nursing home can't require a minimum entrance fee if your care is paid for by Medicare or Medicaid.
- For people seeking admission to the nursing home, the nursing home must tell you (both orally and in writing) and also display written information about how to apply for and use Medicare and Medicaid benefits.
- The nursing home must also provide information on how to get a refund if you paid for an item or service, but because of Medicare and Medicaid eligibility rules, it's now considered covered.

Manage Your Money: You have the right to manage your own money or to choose someone you trust to do this for you. In addition:
- If you deposit your money with the nursing home or ask them to hold or account for your money, you must sign a written statement saying you want them to do this.
- The nursing home must allow you access to your bank accounts, cash, and other financial records.
- The nursing home must have a system that ensures full accounting for your funds and can't combine your funds with the nursing home's funds.

- The nursing home must protect your funds from any loss by providing an acceptable protection, such as buying a surety bond.
- If a resident with a fund dies, the nursing home must return the funds with a final accounting to the person or court handling the resident's estate within 30 days.

Get Proper Privacy, Property, and Living Arrangements: You have the following rights:
- To keep and use your personal belongings and property as long as they don't interfere with the rights, health, or safety of others.
- To have private visits.
- To make and get private phone calls.
- To have privacy in sending and getting mail and email.
- To have the nursing home protect your property from theft.
- To share a room with your spouse if you both live in the same nursing home (if you both agree to do so).
- The nursing home has to notify you before your room or your roommate is changed and should take your preferences into account.
- To review the nursing home's health and fire safety inspection results.

Spend Time with Visitors: You have the following rights:
- To spend private time with visitors.
- To have visitors at any time, as long as you wish to see them, as long as the visit does not interfere with the provision of care and privacy rights of other residents.
- To see any person who gives you help with your health, social, legal, or other services may at any time. This includes your doctor, a representative from the health department, and your Long-Term Care Ombudsman, among others.

Get Social Services: The nursing home must provide you with any needed social services, including the following:
- Counseling.
- Help solving problems with other residents.
- Help in contacting legal and financial professionals.

- Discharge planning.

Leave the Nursing Home:
- Leaving for visits: If your health allows, and your doctor agrees, you can spend time away from the nursing home visiting family or friends during the day or overnight, called a "leave of absence." Talk to the nursing home staff a few days ahead of time so the staff has time to prepare your medicines and write your instructions. Caution: If your nursing home care is covered by certain health insurance, you may not be able to leave for visits without losing your coverage.
- Moving out: Living in a nursing home is your choice. You can choose to move to another place. However, the nursing home may have a policy that requires you to tell them before you plan to leave. If you don't, you may have to pay an extra fee.

Have Protection Against Unfair Transfer or Discharge: You can't be sent to another nursing home, or made to leave the nursing home, unless any of the following are true:
- It's necessary for the welfare, health, or safety of you or others.
- Your health has improved to the point that nursing home care is no longer necessary.
- The nursing home hasn't been paid for services you got.
- The nursing home closes.

You have the following rights:
- You have the right to appeal a transfer or discharge to the State.
- The nursing home can't make you leave if you're waiting to get Medicaid.
- Except in emergencies, nursing homes must give a 30-day written notice of their plan and reason to discharge or transfer you.
- The nursing home has to safely and orderly transfer or discharge you and give you proper notice of bed-hold and/or readmission requirements.

Form or Participate in Resident Groups: You have a right to form or participate in a resident group to discuss issues and concerns about the nursing home's policies and operations. Most homes have such groups, often called "resident councils." The home must give you meeting space and must listen to and act upon grievances and recommendations of the group.

Have Your Family and Friends Involved: Family and friends can help make sure you get good quality care. They can visit and get to know the staff and the nursing home's rules. Family members and legal guardians may meet with the families of other residents and may participate in family councils, if one exists. Family members can help with your care plan with your permission. If a family member or friend is your legal guardian, he or she has the right to look at all medical records about you and make important decisions on your behalf.

References

https://downloads.cms.gov/medicare/Your_Resident_Rights_and_Protections_section.pdf

APPENDIX C: Mealtime

Reality
Every meal is a coordinated effort of kitchen, nursing and housekeeping staffs. The process is routine, yet it is an interruption of all other resident activities.

Responsibilities
Kitchen personnel are charged with having meal trays ready as quickly as nursing staff can serve them but no sooner. Food will not reach the residents at optimal temperature and presentation if trays sit, waiting to be distributed.

Nurses and nurse's aides assure that residents eating in the dining room are sitting at their assigned seats at the specified mealtime. Most residents need assistance to get out of bed and more help to get fully dressed and groomed (an occasional robe is allowed at breakfast). Additionally, residents need assistance to find their hearing aids, eyeglasses, dentures, splints, braces, canes, walkers and wheelchairs. Many residents require further help to transfer into their wheelchairs and then a push to the dining room. The remaining few who can walk independently will need reminders, directions and redirections to find the dining room and their assigned seats.

To a visitor this move toward the dining room resembles a mass migration. To the staff the routine is more like running a marathon at sprinter's speed.

Standards require the presence of a licensed nurse in the dining room during meals. He/she oversees the tray line to guarantee each resident receives the correct food—special diets, food preferences, allergies and fluid restrictions. They also supervise staff, oversee residents and are immediately available for emergencies such as choking.

A vibrant dining room is alive with interaction between residents and staff, residents talking or signaling to each other and exchanges between staff members.

Alert residents enjoy mealtime conversations with their peers. It is worrisome for an independent resident to be seated with someone who cannot speak, may be confused, or needs help to eat. It is equally disturbing for one with limited physical dexterity to be seated at such a table. This resident's spills and messy eating cause personal embarrassment and sometimes resistance to eating. If a messy diner is seated with other messy diners the problem is resolved.

Bibs are a convenience for residents having difficulty eating. Sometimes a poor grip, tremors and poor eyesight lead to spills and dropped food. A resident has a right to refuse a bib, but most agree that removing the bib is easier than changing clothes.

A housekeeping presence is essential for rapid response to all manner of accidents. Delayed response increases the risk of falls, unpleasant odors and sanitary issues. Housekeepers face a cleanup job of huge proportions at meal's end when the dining room exodus is complete.

Staffing

A well-organized dining room can cascade into chaos with a slight glitch. The most difficult to overcome is short staffing. Because staffing for the kitchen, nursing and housekeeping is usually minimal, any absenteeism guarantees a slowdown and predictable trouble.

If the kitchen is missing one person, trays may be delayed. Working short of nurse's aides means residents arrive in the dining room late or are simply relegated to eat in their rooms; their trays will need to be retrieved from the serving line and delivered to their rooms. Fewer staff in the dining room means those residents receive their trays more slowly. Complaints and problems arise as hungry residents become uncomfortable or tired of waiting and simply want to get back to their rooms.

Room Trays

Residents eating in their rooms require the same assistance and oversight as those in the dining room. Sometimes their needs are even greater, yet most of the nursing staff is dispatched to the dining room. Residents eating in their rooms are not visible. It is easier to let them wait for care than to dispatch employees from the dining room where working with fewer employees creates havoc.

Problems encountered by residents eating in their rooms include: trays placed in rooms until someone is available to set up or feed the resident; when staff returns the hot food is cold and the ice cream melted; food may be put out of reach to prevent burns from hot liquids, choking, or to avoid a mess when a weak, confused resident tries to eat; trays may be placed on over-bed tables and slid in front of residents without offering assistance (the resident may be unable to ask for help). The staff member may have every intention of returning, but there are others needing the same help. Additionally, residents confined to the bed will need to be repositioned to an upright sitting position, safe for eating. The effort often requires two staff members.

Food Costs

Each facility has a food budget, which determines how much the Food Service Supervisor (FSS) can spend on meals, snacks and supplemental feedings. The amount is set as a food cost per resident per day. The cost is not allotted to individual residents, rather it is an averaged amount for all residents in the building. In 2017 the average food cost per resident per day ranged from $4.75 to $7.00.

The Registered Dietician plans the monthly meal menu to accommodate the budgeted amount. The FSS is expected to stay within the per resident per day allowance when buying food. Most purchases are made from contracted national food distributors. A typical food contract originates in the facility's distant corporate office.

Simple nutritional snacks and supplements recommended by the RD can become an issue because of the cost. A physician's order may be necessary to justify supplemental feedings for midmorning, midafternoon and bedtime.

Most facilities avoid serving a bedtime snack to all residents by scheduling meals with no more than fourteen hours elapsing between the evening meal and breakfast. Standards still require that some snacks are available on the nursing units after the kitchen closes for the evening. However, costs and the idea that employees will eat them dominate reasons for limiting snack foods on the nursing units. The kitchen is usually locked and food is not accessible to nurses during the late evening and night shift.

ACKNOWLEDGMENTS

I am indebted to my family, Sam, Kole, and Sally. They never quit asking, "So how's the book coming?" Bill, of course. He was my harshest critic, but always offered sage contributions for each shortcoming . . . I welcomed and included each one. Their reading, intervention and cumulative push helped finalized the book.

Any recognition of my writing partners, Rose Hall and Rhonda Wiley-Jones, falls far short of their contributions. Each revision evoked Rose's reminder, "Don't let perfection get in the way of progress." Yet, she remained long-suffering to the end. Rhonda taught me about the craft of writing and the patience to rewrite. Both read far more than any normal interest in nursing homes might carry them and I am grateful.

Skye Alexander's Dietert Center class endured my unpolished effort and offered wise counsel for improvements. The group shared their professional insight with good cheer and my first literary effort is better because of them. Skye's final review, edits and print suggestions moved the effort toward a more professional product.

Richard Weathermon (Mother's beloved Dick) and Jean helped with the final draft.

Fellow writers prodded me with reminders of the need for nursing home information: Garland O'Quinn, George Fischer, Helen Nourse and many others. I took the reminders to indicate confidence in the book's content, so each became a motivational boost. Family and friends, who read, judged content and offered suggestions include Loke Lovett, Heidi Faesler, Karen Moos and Janie Fitzgerald.

At the monthly D'Hanis retired teachers' luncheons, I listened to long-time neighbors bemoan the fate of mutual friends facing the uncertainties of failing health. The need for long-term-care loomed as a possibility for each of us . . . perhaps our own need or maybe a loved one. These friendships lent urgency to my project.

None of this would have been possible without the residents and their families who taught me so much. Each one enriched my life and my writing. I attempted to capture the significance of their lives, but in all instances my narratives seem insufficient. Nevertheless, I hope the reader is able to appreciate their wisdom, character and contributions.

ABOUT THE AUTHOR

Frances Lovett, RN, is the person you would want to have as a guide and mentor if you have a loved one already living in a nursing home or will soon need nursing home care.

The author is a 1961 graduate of Hendrick Memorial Hospital School of Nursing in Abilene, Texas. She practiced her profession in Oklahoma, Kansas, South Carolina, and Texas. Her employment ran the gamut of hospital specialty areas before partnering with a fellow nurse to establish a privately owned home health agency serving mostly Medicare patients.

Frances Lovett's early nursing home experience began as part time consulting intertwined with hospital and home health practice. The last thirty years of her career were devoted to nursing home care. Positions included staff nurse, supervisor, nurse manager, and Medicare coordinator. She was director of nursing at several facilities. As a certified wound care nurse she consulted in facilities throughout Texas for prevention and treatment of skin ulcers. Later practice included financial auditing, legal consulting and expert testimony for nursing home litigation.

As an employee she gained insight into how budgets and financing impact care through work at the Veterans Administration, state institutions, local governments, private ownership, religious affiliations and multiple corporations. As an employer Frances Lovett shouldered accountability for care and finances.

As a healthcare consumer and caregiver Frances Lovett shepherded her mother through nursing home care, her son through a liver transplant, and her husband through a terminal illness. She is a breast cancer survivor.

www.ingramcontent.com/pod-product-compliance
Lightning Source LLC
Chambersburg PA
CBHW052311220526
45472CB00001B/62